The Mediterranean Diet Recipe Book

2 Books in 1: 200 + Easy Recipes to Start a Heathy Lifestyle!!! Taste the Mediterranean Meals Flavors and Follow the Guide for Beginners Inside!

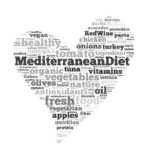

By

Alexander Sandler

TABLE OF CONTENT

PART I: INTRODUCTION

Today, many people, especially teenagers, fill their plates with pizza, white bread, refined sugar, and processed food with lots of preservatives.

But analysis and research on processed foods such as frozen food, white bread, and carbonated beverages have led to surprising facts. Habitual consumption of these foods can tax the body. Excessive consumption can lead to high insulin production. This can cause diabetes, obesity, and coronary artery malfunction.

The reality of animal fats is not much different. Saturated fats in these foods can hurt our bodies. It causes the accumulation of extra fat in our body and disturbs our body mass index. Saturated fat in animal products like milk and butter increases lousy cholesterol or LDL. In short, it can damage the health of the coronary arteries.

In this technologically advanced society, when we can accomplish our tasks with little effort, physical activities are negligible. Poor health conveniently comes into play. It becomes essential to switch to a healthier diet that meets our body's nutritional needs while keeping us full.

The Mediterranean diet can do this. It is an eating pattern that overflows with whole grains, a plant-based diet in which olive oil is a fat source. This diet has no room for processed foods loaded with sugar or artificial sweeteners. The low amount of fat keeps your heart healthy and provides both essential nutrients and agility. Give it a try, and you won't look back. You will leap into a healthy future.

I wish you all the best in healthy eating.

START TO GET FAMILIAR WITH THE MEDITERRANEAN DIET

When you read the word "Mediterranean," you tend to think of the sea. This brings to mind seafood. The diet has its roots in the Mediterranean basin, a land that has historically been called a powerhouse of societal evolution. This area of the Nile Valley was good land for the peoples of the East and West. The frequent interaction of people from different regions and cultures had a significant effect on customs, languages, religion, and outlook and positively impacted lifestyles. This integration and cultural clash further influenced eating habits.

Looking at the Mediterranean diet's food content, one can see the reflection of different cultures and classes. Bread, wine, and oil reflect agriculture; lettuce, mushrooms, and mallow further complement this. There is a slight preference for meat but much preference for fish and seafood. This shows the greedy nature of the people of Rome. Here we also have the Germanic flavor of pork with garden vegetables. Beer was made from grains.

The food culture of bread, wine, and oil went beyond the Germanic and Christian Roman culture and entered the borders of the Arabs. The reason was their existence on the southern shore of the Mediterranean. Their food culture was unique because of the variety of leafy vegetables they grew. They had eggplant, spinach, sugarcane, and fruits such as oranges, citrus, lemon, and pomegranate. This influenced the cooking style of the Latinos and influenced their recipes.

The great geographical event that is the discovery of America by Europeans has a great additional impact on the Mediterranean diet. This event added several new foods such as beans, potatoes, tomatoes, chili peppers, and peppers. The tomato, the red plant, was first ornamental and then considered edible. It then became an essential part of the Mediterranean diet.

Historical analysis of the Mediterranean diet shows how the Egyptians' diet at the discovery of America gave us the Mediterranean diet of today. The Mediterranean diet's nutritional model is intimately linked to the Mediterranean people, lifestyle, and history.

Some established health and cultural platforms, such as UNESCO, define the Mediterranean diet, explaining the meaning of the word "diet," which comes from the word "data," meaning lifestyle or way of life. It focuses on food from landscape to table, covering cooking, harvesting, processing, preparation, fishing, cooking, and a specific form of consumption.

There is a variation in the Mediterranean diet in different countries due to ethnic and cultural differences, other religions, and economic disparity. According to the description and recommendation of dieticians and food experts, the Mediterranean diet has the proportion of the following food. In grains, there are whole grains and legumes. For fats, olive oil is the primary source. Onion, garlic, tomatoes, leafy greens, and peppers are the main vegetables. Fresh fruit is the main one in snacks and desserts. Eggs, milk, yogurt, and other dairy products are taken moderately. Foods such as red meat, processed foods, and refined sugar are handled as little as possible.

This diet has a fat ratio of 25% to 35% in calories, and saturated fat never exceeds 8%. As for oil, alternatives are depending on the region. In central and northern Italy, butter and lard are commonly used in cooking. Olive is used primarily for snacks and salad dressing.

This diet reflects Crete's dietary pattern, the rest of Greece, and much of Italy in the early 1960s. It gained widespread recognition in the 1990s. There is an irony to the Mediterranean diet. Although people who live in this region tend to consume a high amount of fat, they enjoy much better cardiovascular health than people in America who consume an equal amount of fat.

The Mediterranean diet tradition offers a cuisine rich in color, taste, flavor, and aroma. Above all, it keeps us closer to nature. It may be simple in appearance, but rich in health and has much to offer that is in no way inferior to any other healthy diet. Some Americans describe the Mediterranean diet as homemade pasta with parmesan sauce and enriched with a few pieces of meat. It includes lots of fresh vegetables with just olive oil drizzled on top. Desserts in this diet include fresh fruit.

An excellent Mediterranean diet does not include soy, canola, or any other refined oil. There is no room for processed meat, refined sugar, white bread, refined grains, white pasta, or pizza dough containing white flour.

This diet features a balanced use of foods with high amounts of fiber, unsaturated fat s, and antioxidants. Besides, there is an approach that prioritizes health by cutting unhealthy animal fats and meat consumption. This way, a balance is achieved between the amount of energy intake and its consumption.

This magical diet is not only a preferred approach to health, with a wide range of magical recipes but also a channel between the most diverse cultures. The inhabitants of this region are children of the earth, and so is their food from the land and soil. It can ensure if consumed rationally, the effectiveness of various bodily functions.

Some well-known health organizations worldwide have designed food pyramids to clarify the most common forms of the Mediterranean region. It has become popular among health activists because people from this region have high life expectancy despite less access to healthcare facilities. It has been stated by the American Heart Association and the American Diabetes Association that the Mediterranean diet lowers the risk of cardiovascular disease and type 2 diabetes. If a Mediterranean diet plan is followed, it can have a lasting effect on health and help reduce and maintain a healthy weight.

THE BENEFITS OF THE MEDITERRANEAN DIET

The Mediterranean diet has gained popularity in medical fields because of its documented benefits for heart health. But, much research has shown that the Mediterranean diet may have a much longer list of health benefits that go beyond the heart. This will review just a few of the many improvements you can experience with your health when you start following the Mediterranean diet.

REDUCES AGE-RELATED MUSCLE AND BONE WEAKNESS

Eating a well-balanced diet that provides a wide range of vitamins and minerals is essential for reducing muscle weakness and bone degradation. This is especially important as you age. Accident-related injuries, such as tripping, falling, or slipping while walking, can cause serious injuries. As you age, this becomes even more concerning because some simple falls can be fatal. Many accidents occur because of weakening muscle mass and loss of bone density. Women, especially those entering the menopausal stage of their lives, are more at risk of severe injuries from accidental falls because estrogen levels decrease significantly during this time—this decrease in estrogen results in a loss of bone muscle mass. Reduced estrogen can also cause bone thinning, which over time develops into osteoporosis.

Maintaining healthy bone mass and muscle agility as you age can be a challenge. When you don't get the proper nutrients to promote healthy bones and muscles, you increase your risk of developing osteoporosis. The Mediterranean diet offers an easy way to meet the dietary needs necessary to improve bone and muscle function.

Antioxidants, vitamins C and K, carotenoids, magnesium, potassium, and phytoestrogens are essential minerals and nutrients for optimal musculoskeletal health. Plant-based foods, unsaturated fats, and whole grains help provide the necessary balance of nutrients that keep bones and muscles healthy. Following a Mediterranean diet can improve and reduce bone loss as you age.

The Mediterranean diet consists of many foods that increase the risk of Alzheimer's, such as processed meats, refined grains like white bread and pasta, and added sugar. Foods that contain dactyl, which is a chemical commonly used in the refining process, increase the buildup of beta-amyloid plaques in the brain. Microwave popcorn, margarine, and butter are some of the most frequently consumed foods that contain this harmful chemical. It's no wonder that Alzheimer's is becoming one of the leading causes of death among Americans.

On the other hand, the Mediterranean diet includes a wide range of foods that have been shown to boost memory and slow cognitive decline. Dark leafy vegetables, fresh berries, extra virgin olive oil, and fresh fish contain vitamins and minerals that can improve brain health. The Mediterranean diet can help you make necessary diet and lifestyle changes that can significantly decrease your risk of Alzheimer's.

The Mediterranean diet encourages improvement in both diet and physical activity. Thanks to these two components are the most important factors that will help you manage the symptoms of diabetes and reduce your risk of developing the condition.

HEART HEALTH AND STROKE RISK REDUCTION

Heart health is strongly influenced by diet. Maintaining healthy cholesterol levels, blood pressure, blood sugar, and staying within a beneficial weight results in optimal heart health. Your diet directly affects each of these components. Those at increased risk are often advised to start on a low-fat diet. A low-fat diet eliminates all fats, including those from oils, nuts, and red meat. Studies have shown that the Mediterranean diet, which includes healthy fats, is more effective at lowering cardiovascular risks than a standard low-fat diet: (that's processed red meat, 2019). This is because the unsaturated fats consumed in the Mediterranean diet lower bad cholesterol levels and increase good cholesterol levels.

The Mediterranean diet emphasizes the importance of daily activity and stress reduction by enjoying quality time with friends and family. Each of these elements, along with eating more plant-based foods, significantly improves heart health and reduces the risk of many heart-related conditions. By increasing your intake of fresh fruits and vegetables and adding regular daily activities, you improve not only your heart health but your overall health.

ADDITIONAL BENEFITS

Aside from the significant benefits to your heart and brain, the Mediterranean diet can significantly improve many other key factors in your life. Since the Mediterranean diet focuses on eating healthy, exercising, and connecting with others, you can see improvements to your mental health, physical health and often feel like you're living a more fulfilling life.

PROTECTS AGAINST CANCER

Many plant-based foods, especially those in the yellow and orange color groups, contain cancer-fighting agents. Increasing the antioxidants consumed by eating fresh fruits and vegetables, and whole grains can protect the body's cells from developing cancer cells. Drinking a glass of red wine also provides cancer-protective compounds.

ENERGY

Following a Mediterranean diet focuses on fueling your body. Other diets focus only on filling your body, and this is often done through empty calories. When your body gets the nutrients it needs, it can function properly, which results in feeling more energized throughout the day. You won't need to rely on sugary drinks, excess caffeine, or sugar-filled energy bars to get you going and keep you moving. You'll feel less weighed down after eating, and that translates into a greater capacity for output.

GET BETTER SLEEP

Sugar and caffeine can cause significant sleep disturbances. Besides, other foods, such as processed foods, can make it harder to get the right amount of sleep. When you eat the right foods, you can see a change in your sleep patterns. Your body will want to rest to recover and properly absorb the vitamins and minerals consumed during the day. Your brain will switch into sleep mode with ease because it has received the vitamins it needs to function correctly. When you get the right amount of sleep, you will, in turn, have more energy the next day, and this can also significantly improve your mood. The Mediterranean diet increases nutrient-dense food consumption and avoids excess sugar and processed foods known to cause sleep problems.

Besides, the Mediterranean diet allows you to maintain a healthy weight, reducing the risk of developing sleep disorders such as sleep apnea. Sleep apnea is common in individuals who are overweight and obese. It causes the airway to become blocked, making it difficult to breathe. This results in not getting enough oxygen when you sleep, which can cause sudden and frequent awakenings during the night.

LONGEVITY

The Mediterranean diet, indeed, helps reduce the risk of many health problems. Its heart, brain, and mood health benefits translate into a longer, more enjoyable life. When you eliminate the risk of developing certain conditions such as cardiovascular disease, diabetes, and dementia, you increase your lifespan. But eliminating these health risks is not the only cause of increased longevity with the Mediterranean diet. Increased physical activity and deep social connection also play a significant role in living a longer life.

CLEAR SKIN

Healthy skin starts on the inside. When you provide your body with healthy foods, it radiates through your skin. The antioxidants in extra virgin olive oil alone are enough to keep your skin young and healthy. But the Mediterranean diet includes many fresh fruits and vegetables that are full of antioxidants. These antioxidants help repair damaged cells in the body and promote the growth of healthy cells. Eating a variety of healthy fats also keeps your skin supple and can protect it from premature aging.

MAINTAINING A HEALTHY WEIGHT

With the Mediterranean diet, you eat mostly whole, fresh foods. Eating more foods rich in vitamins, minerals, and nutrients is essential to maintaining a healthy weight. The diet is easy to stick to, and there are no calorie restrictions to follow strictly. This makes it a highly sustainable plan for those who want to lose weight or maintain a healthy weight. Keep in mind; this is not an option to lose weight fast. This is a lifestyle that will allow you to maintain optimal health for years, not just a few months.

Breakfast

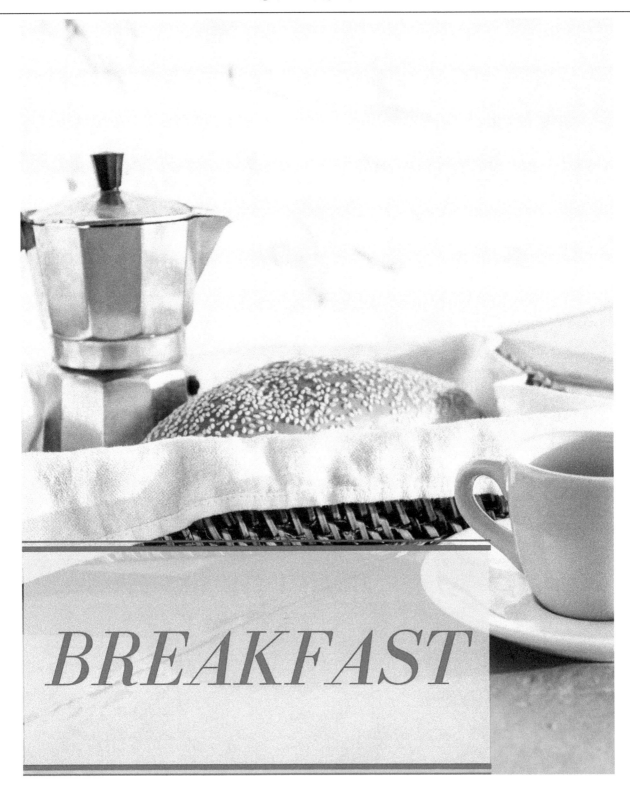

BREAKFAST

1) CAULIFLOWER FRITTERS AND HUMMUS

Cooking Time: 15 Minutes   **Servings: 4**

Ingredients:

- ✓ 2 (15 oz) cans chickpeas, divided
- ✓ 2 1/2 tbsp olive oil, divided, plus more for frying
- ✓ 1 cup onion, chopped, about 1/2 a small onion
- ✓ 2 tbsp garlic, minced
- ✓ 2 cups cauliflower, cut into small pieces, about 1/2 a large head
- ✓ 1/2 tsp salt
- ✓ black pepper
- ✓ Topping:
- ✓ Hummus, of choice
- ✓ Green onion, diced

Directions:

- ❖ Preheat oven to 400°F
- ❖ Rinse and drain 1 can of the chickpeas, place them on a paper towel to dry off well
- ❖ Then place the chickpeas into a large bowl, removing the loose skins that come off, and toss with 1 tbsp of olive oil, spread the chickpeas onto a large pan (being careful not to over-crowd them) and sprinkle with salt and pepper
- ❖ Bake for 20 minutes, then stir, and then bake an additional 5-10 minutes until very crispy
- ❖ Once the chickpeas are roasted, transfer them to a large food processor and process until broken down and crumble - Don't over process them and turn it into flour, as you need to have some texture. Place the mixture into a small bowl, set aside
- ❖ In a large pan over medium-high heat, add the remaining 1 1/2 tbsp of olive oil
- ❖ Once heated, add in the onion and garlic, cook until lightly golden brown, about 2 minutes. Then add in the chopped cauliflower, cook for an additional 2 minutes, until the cauliflower is golden
- ❖ Turn the heat down to low and cover the pan, cook until the cauliflower is fork tender and the onions are golden brown and caramelized, stirring often, about 3-5 minutes
- ❖ Transfer the cauliflower mixture to the food processor, drain and rinse the remaining can of chickpeas and add them into the food processor, along with the salt and a pinch of pepper. Blend until smooth, and the mixture starts to ball, stop to scrape down the sides as needed
- ❖ Transfer the cauliflower mixture into a large bowl and add in 1/2 cup of the roasted chickpea crumbs (you won't use all of the crumbs, but it is easier to break them down when you have a larger amount.), stir until well combined
- ❖ In a large bowl over medium heat, add in enough oil to lightly cover the bottom of a large pan
- ❖ Working in batches, cook the patties until golden brown, about 2-3 minutes, flip and cook again
- ❖ Distribute among the container, placing parchment paper in between the fritters. Store in the fridge for 2-3 days
- ❖ To Serve: Heat through in the oven at 350F for 5-8 minutes. Top with hummus, green onion and enjoy!
- ❖ Recipe Notes: Don't add too much oil while frying the fritter or they will end up soggy. Use only enough to cover the pan. Use a fork while frying and resist the urge to flip them every minute to see if they are golden

Nutrition: Calories:333;Total Carbohydrates: 45g;Total Fat: 13g;Protein: 14g

2) ITALIAN BREAKFAST SAUSAGE AND BABY POTATOES WITH VEGETABLES

Cooking Time: 30 Minutes   **Servings: 4**

Ingredients:

- ✓ 1 lbs sweet Italian sausage links, sliced on the bias (diagonal)
- ✓ 2 cups baby potatoes, halved
- ✓ 2 cups broccoli florets
- ✓ 1 cup onions cut to 1-inch chunks
- ✓ 2 cups small mushrooms -half or quarter the large ones for uniform size
- ✓ 1 cup baby carrots
- ✓ 2 tbsp olive oil
- ✓ 1/2 tsp garlic powder
- ✓ 1/2 tsp Italian seasoning
- ✓ 1 tsp salt
- ✓ 1/2 tsp pepper

Directions:

- ❖ Preheat the oven to 400 degrees F
- ❖ In a large bowl, add the baby potatoes, broccoli florets, onions, small mushrooms, and baby carrots
- ❖ Add in the olive oil, salt, pepper, garlic powder and Italian seasoning and toss to evenly coat
- ❖ Spread the vegetables onto a sheet pan in one even layer
- ❖ Arrange the sausage slices on the pan over the vegetables
- ❖ Bake for 30 minutes – make sure to sake halfway through to prevent sticking
- ❖ Allow to cool
- ❖ Distribute the Italian sausages and vegetables among the containers and store in the fridge for 2-3 days
- ❖ To Serve: Reheat in the microwave for 1-2 minutes, or until heated through and enjoy!
- ❖ Recipe Notes: If you would like crispier potatoes, place them on the pan and bake for 15 minutes before adding the other ingredients to the pan.

Nutrition: Calories:321;Total Fat: 16g;Total Carbs: 23g;Fiber: 4g;Protein: 22g

3) BREAKFAST GREEK QUINOA BOWL

Cooking Time: 20 Minutes   **Servings: 6**

Ingredients:

- ✓ 12 eggs
- ✓ ¼ cup plain Greek yogurt
- ✓ 1 tsp onion powder
- ✓ 1 tsp granulated garlic
- ✓ ½ tsp salt
- ✓ ½ tsp pepper
- ✓ 1 tsp olive oil
- ✓ 1 (5 oz) bag baby spinach
- ✓ 1 pint cherry tomatoes, halved
- ✓ 1 cup feta cheese
- ✓ 2 cups cooked quinoa

Directions:

- ❖ In a large bowl whisk together eggs, Greek yogurt, onion powder, granulated garlic, salt, and pepper, set aside
- ❖ In a large skillet, heat olive oil and add spinach, cook the spinach until it is slightly wilted, about 3-4 minutes
- ❖ Add in cherry tomatoes, cook until tomatoes are softened, 4 minutes
- ❖ Stir in egg mixture and cook until the eggs are set, about 7-9 minutes, stir in the eggs as they cook to scramble
- ❖ Once the eggs have set stir in the feta and quinoa, cook until heated through
- ❖ Distribute evenly among the containers, store for 2-3 days
- ❖ To serve: Reheat in the microwave for 30 seconds to 1 minute or heated through

Nutrition: Calories:357;Total Carbohydrates: ;Total Fat: 20g;Protein: 23g

4) EGG, HAM WITH CHEESE FREEZER SANDWICHES

Cooking Time: 20 Minutes   **Servings:** 6

Ingredients:

- ✓ Cooking spray or oil to grease the baking dish
- ✓ 7 large eggs
- ✓ ½ cup low-fat (2%) milk
- ✓ ½ tsp garlic powder
- ✓ ½ tsp onion powder
- ✓ 1 tbsp Dijon mustard
- ✓ ½ tsp honey
- ✓ 6 whole-wheat English muffins
- ✓ 6 slices thinly sliced prosciutto
- ✓ 6 slices Swiss cheese

Directions:

- ❖ Preheat the oven to 375°F. Lightly oil or spray an 8-by--inch glass or ceramic baking dish with cooking spray.
- ❖ In a large bowl, whisk together the eggs, milk, garlic powder, and onion powder. Pour the mixture into the baking dish and bake for minutes, until the eggs are set and no longer jiggling. Cool.
- ❖ While the eggs are baking, mix the mustard and honey in a small bowl. Lay out the English muffin halves to start assembly.
- ❖ When the eggs are cool, use a biscuit cutter or drinking glass about the same size as the English muffin diameter to cut 6 egg circles. Divide the leftover egg scraps evenly to be added to each sandwich.
- ❖ Spread ½ tsp of honey mustard on each of the bottom English muffin halves. Top each with 1 slice of prosciutto, 1 egg circle and scraps, 1 slice of cheese, and the top half of the muffin.
- ❖ Wrap each sandwich tightly in foil.
- ❖ STORAGE: Store tightly wrapped sandwiches in the freezer for up to 1 month. To reheat, remove the foil, place the sandwich on a microwave-safe plate, and wrap with a damp paper towel. Microwave on high for 1½ minutes, flip over, and heat again for another 1½ minutes. Because cooking time can vary greatly between microwaves, you may need to experiment with a few sandwiches before you find the perfect amount of time to heat the whole item through.

Nutrition: Total calories: 361; Total fat: 17g; Saturated fat: 7g; Sodium: 953mg; Carbohydrates: 26g; Fiber: 3g; Protein: 24g

5) HEALTHY SALAD ZUCCHINI KALE TOMATO

Cooking Time: 20 Minutes   **Servings:** 4

Ingredients:

- ✓ 1 lb kale, chopped
- ✓ 2 tbsp fresh parsley, chopped
- ✓ 1 tbsp vinegar
- ✓ 1/2 cup can tomato, crushed
- ✓ 1 tsp paprika
- ✓ 1 cup zucchini, cut into cubes
- ✓ 1 cup grape tomatoes, halved
- ✓ 2 tbsp olive oil
- ✓ 1 onion, chopped
- ✓ 1 leek, sliced
- ✓ Pepper
- ✓ Salt

Directions:

- ❖ Add oil into the inner pot of instant pot and set the pot on sauté mode.
- ❖ Add leek and onion and sauté for 5 minutes.
- ❖ Add kale and remaining ingredients and stir well.
- ❖ Seal pot with lid and cook on high for 15 minutes.
- ❖ Once done, allow to release pressure naturally for 10 minutes then release remaining using quick release. Remove lid.
- ❖ Stir and serve.

Nutrition: Calories: 162;Fat: 3 g;Carbohydrates: 22.2 g;Sugar: 4.8 g;Protein: 5.2 g;Cholesterol: 0 mg

6) CHEESE WITH CAULIFLOWER FRITTATA AND PEPPERS

Cooking Time: 30 Minutes   **Servings: 6**

Ingredients:

- ✓ 10 eggs
- ✓ 1 seeded and chopped bell pepper
- ✓ ½ cup grated Parmigiano-Reggiano
- ✓ ½ cup milk, skim
- ✓ ½ tsp cayenne pepper
- ✓ 1 pound cauliflower, floret
- ✓ ½ tsp saffron
- ✓ 2 tbsp chopped chives
- ✓ Salt and black pepper as desired

Directions:

- ❖ Prepare your oven by setting the temperature to 370 degrees Fahrenheit. You should also grease a skillet suitable for the oven.
- ❖ In a medium-sized bowl, add the milk and eggs. Whisk them until they are frothy.
- ❖ Sprinkle the grated Parmigiano-Reggiano cheese into the frothy mixture and fold the ingredients together.
- ❖ Pour in the salt, saffron, cayenne pepper, and black pepper and gently stir.
- ❖ Add in the chopped bell pepper and gently stir until the ingredients are fully incorporated.
- ❖ Pour the egg mixture into the skillet and cook on medium heat over your stovetop for 4 minutes.
- ❖ Steam the cauliflower florets in a pan. To do this, add ½ inch of water and ½ tsp sea salt. Pour in the cauliflower and cover for 3 to 8 minutes. Drain any extra water.
- ❖ Add the cauliflower into the mixture and gently stir.
- ❖ Set the skillet into the preheated oven and turn your timer to 13 minutes. Once the mixture is golden brown in the middle, remove the frittata from the oven.
- ❖ Set your skillet aside for a couple of minutes so it can cool.
- ❖ Slice and garnish with chives before you serve.

Nutrition: calories: 207, fats: grams, carbohydrates: 8 grams, protein: 17 grams.

7) AVOCADO KALE OMELETTE

Cooking Time: 5 Minutes   **Servings: 1**

Ingredients:

- ✓ 2 eggs
- ✓ 1 tsp milk
- ✓ 2 tsp olive oil
- ✓ 1 cup kale (chopped)
- ✓ 1 tbsp lime juice
- ✓ 1 tbsp cilantro (chopped)
- ✓ 1 tsp sunflower seeds
- ✓ Pinch of red pepper (crushed)
- ✓ ¼ avocado (sliced)
- ✓ sea salt or plain salt
- ✓ freshly ground black pepper

Directions:

- ❖ Toss all the Ingredients: (except eggs and milk) to make the kale salad.
- ❖ Beat the eggs and milk in a bowl.
- ❖ Heat oil in a pan over medium heat. Then pour in the egg mixture and cook it until the bottom settles. Cook for 2 minutes and then flip it over and further cook for 20 seconds.
- ❖ Finally, put the Omelette in containers.
- ❖ Top the Omelette with the kale salad.
- ❖ Serve warm.

Nutrition: Calories: 399, Total Fat: 28.8g, Saturated Fat: 6.2, Cholesterol: 328 mg, Sodium: 162 mg, Total Carbohydrate: 25.2g, Dietary Fiber: 6.3 g, Total Sugars: 9 g, Protein: 15.8 g, Vitamin D: 31 mcg, Calcium: 166 mg, Iron: 4 mg, Potassium: 980 mg

8) BREAKFAST WITH MEDITERRANEAN-STYLE BURRITO

Cooking Time: 5 Minutes   **Servings:** 6

Ingredients:

- ✓ 9 eggs whole
- ✓ 6 tortillas whole 10 inch, regular or sun-dried tomato
- ✓ 3 tbsp sun-dried tomatoes, chopped
- ✓ 1/2 cup feta cheese I use light/low-fat feta
- ✓ 2 cups baby spinach washed and dried
- ✓ 3 tbsp black olives, sliced
- ✓ 3/4 cup refried beans, canned
- ✓ Garnish:
- ✓ Salsa

Directions:

- ❖ Spray a medium frying pan with non- stick spray, add the eggs and scramble and toss for about 5 minutes, or until eggs are no longer liquid
- ❖ Add in the spinach, black olives, sun-dried tomatoes and continue to stir and toss until no longer wet
- ❖ Add in the feta cheese and cover, cook until cheese is melted
- ❖ Add 2 tbsp of refried beans to each tortilla
- ❖ Top with egg mixture, dividing evenly between all burritos, and wrap
- ❖ Frying in a pan until lightly browned
- ❖ Allow to cool completely before slicing
- ❖ Wrap the slices in plastic wrap and then aluminum foil and place in the freezer for up to 2 months or fridge for 2 days
- ❖ To Serve: Remove the aluminum foil and plastic wrap, and microwave for 2 minutes, then allow to rest for 30 seconds, enjoy! Enjoy hot with salsa and fruit

Nutrition: Calories:252;Total Carbohydrates: 21g;Total Fat: 11g;Protein: 14g |

9) SHAKSHUKA AND FETA

Cooking Time: 40 Minutes   **Servings:** 4-6

Ingredients:

- ✓ 6 large eggs
- ✓ 3 tbsp extra-virgin olive oil
- ✓ 1 large onion, halved and thinly sliced
- ✓ 1 large red bell pepper, seeded and thinly sliced
- ✓ 3 garlic cloves, thinly sliced
- ✓ 1 tsp ground cumin
- ✓ 1 tsp sweet paprika
- ✓ ⅛ tsp cayenne, or to taste
- ✓ 1 (28-ounce) can whole plum tomatoes with juices, coarsely chopped
- ✓ ¾ tsp salt, more as needed
- ✓ ¼ tsp black pepper, more as needed
- ✓ 5 oz feta cheese, crumbled, about 1 1/4 cups
- ✓ To Serve:
- ✓ Chopped cilantro
- ✓ Hot sauce

Directions:

- ❖ Preheat oven to 375 degrees F
- ❖ In a large skillet over medium-low heat, add the oil
- ❖ Once heated, add the onion and bell pepper, cook gently until very soft, about 20 minutes
- ❖ Add in the garlic and cook until tender, 1 to 2 minutes, then stir in cumin, paprika and cayenne, and cook 1 minute
- ❖ Pour in tomatoes, season with 3/4 tsp salt and 1/4 tsp pepper, simmer until tomatoes have thickened, about 10 minutes
- ❖ Then stir in crumbled feta
- ❖ Gently crack eggs into skillet over tomatoes, season with salt and pepper
- ❖ Transfer skillet to oven
- ❖ Bake until eggs have just set, 7 to 10 minutes
- ❖ Allow to cool and distribute among the containers, store in the fridge for 2-3 days
- ❖ To Serve: Reheat in the oven at 360 degrees F for 5 minutes or until heated through

Nutrition: Calories:337;Carbs: 17g;Total Fat: 25g;Protein

10) SPINACH, FETA WITH EGG BREAKFAST QUESADILLAS

Cooking Time: 15 Minutes   **Servings: 5**

Ingredients:

- 8 eggs (optional)
- 2 tsp olive oil
- 1 red bell pepper
- 1/2 red onion
- 1/4 cup milk
- 4 handfuls of spinach leaves
- 1 1/2 cup mozzarella cheese
- 5 sun-dried tomato tortillas
- 1/2 cup feta
- 1/4 tsp salt
- 1/4 tsp pepper
- Spray oil

Directions:

- In a large non-stick pan over medium heat, add the olive oil
- Once heated, add the bell pepper and onion, cook for 4-5 minutes until soft
- In the meantime, whisk together the eggs, milk, salt and pepper in a bowl
- Add in the egg/milk mixture into the pan with peppers and onions, stirring frequently, until eggs are almost cooked through
- Add in the spinach and feta, fold into the eggs, stirring until spinach is wilted and eggs are cooked through
- Remove the eggs from heat and plate
- Spray a separate large non-stick pan with spray oil, and place over medium heat
- Add the tortilla, on one half of the tortilla, spread about ½ cup of the egg mixture
- Top the eggs with around ⅓ cup of shredded mozzarella cheese
- Fold the second half of the tortilla over, then cook for 2 minutes, or until golden brown
- Flip and cook for another minute until golden brown
- Allow the quesadilla to cool completely, divide among the container, store for 2 days or wrap in plastic wrap and foil, and freeze for up to 2 months
- To Serve: Reheat in oven at 375 for 3-5 minutes or until heated through

Nutrition: (1/2 quesadilla): Calories:213;Total Fat: 11g;Total Carbs: 15g;Protein: 15g

11) BREAKFAST COBBLER

Cooking Time: 12 Minutes   **Servings: 4**

Ingredients:

- 2 lbs apples, cut into chunks
- 1 1/2 cups water
- 1/4 tsp nutmeg
- 1 1/2 tsp cinnamon
- 1/2 cup dry buckwheat
- 1/2 cup dates, chopped
- Pinch of ground ginger

Directions:

- Spray instant pot from inside with cooking spray.
- Add all ingredients into the instant pot and stir well.
- Seal pot with a lid and select manual and set timer for 12 minutes.
- Once done, release pressure using quick release. Remove lid.
- Stir and serve.

Nutrition: Calories: 195;Fat: 0.9 g;Carbohydrates: 48.3 g;Sugar: 25.8 g;Protein: 3.3 g;Cholesterol: 0 mg

13) EGG-TOPPED QUINOA BOWL AND KALE

Cooking Time: 5 Minutes   **Servings: 2**

Ingredients:

- 1-ounce pancetta, chopped
- 1 bunch kale, sliced
- ½ cup cherry tomatoes, halved
- 1 tsp red wine vinegar
- 1 cup cooked quinoa
- 1 tsp olive oil
- 2 eggs
- 1/3 cup avocado, sliced
- sea salt or plain salt
- fresh black pepper

Directions:

- Start by heating pancetta in a skillet until golden brown. Add in kale and further cook for 2 minutes.
- Then, stir in tomatoes, vinegar, and salt and remove from heat.
- Now, divide this mixture into 2 bowls, add avocado to both, and then set aside.
- Finally, cook both the eggs and top each bowl with an egg.
- Serve hot with toppings of your choice.

Nutrition: Calories: 547, Total Fat: 22., Saturated Fat: 5.3, Cholesterol: 179 mg, Sodium: 412 mg, Total Carbohydrate: 62.5 g, Dietary Fiber: 8.6 g, Total Sugars: 1.7 g, Protein: 24.7 g, Vitamin D: 15 mcg, Calcium: 117 mg, Iron: 6 mg, Potassium: 1009 mg

14) STRAWBERRY GREEK COLD YOGURT

Cooking Time: 2-4 Hours   **Servings: 5**

Ingredients:

- ✓ 3 cups plain Greek low-fat yogurt
- ✓ 1 cup sugar
- ✓ ¼ cup lemon juice, freshly squeezed
- ✓ 2 tsp vanilla
- ✓ 1/8 tsp salt
- ✓ 1 cup strawberries, sliced

Directions:

- ❖ In a medium-sized bowl, add yogurt, lemon juice, sugar, vanilla, and salt.
- ❖ Whisk the whole mixture well.
- ❖ Freeze the yogurt mix in a 2-quart ice cream maker according to the given instructions.
- ❖ During the final minute, add the sliced strawberries.
- ❖ Transfer the yogurt to an airtight container.
- ❖ Place in the freezer for 2-4 hours.
- ❖ Remove from the freezer and allow it to stand for 5-15 minutes.
- ❖ Serve and enjoy!

Nutrition: Calories: 251, Total Fat: 0.5 g, Saturated Fat: 0.1 g, Cholesterol: 3 mg, Sodium: 130 mg, Total Carbohydrate: 48.7 g, Dietary Fiber: 0.6 g, Total Sugars: 47.3 g, Protein: 14.7 g, Vitamin D: 1 mcg, Calcium: 426 mg, Iron: 0 mg, Potassium: 62 mg

15) PEACH ALMOND OATMEAL

Cooking Time: 10 Minutes   **Servings: 2**

Ingredients:

- ✓ 1 cup unsweetened almond milk
- ✓ 2 cups of water
- ✓ 1 cup oats
- ✓ 2 peaches, diced
- ✓ Pinch of salt

Directions:

- ❖ Spray instant pot from inside with cooking spray.
- ❖ Add all ingredients into the instant pot and stir well.
- ❖ Seal pot with a lid and select manual and set timer for 10 minutes.
- ❖ Once done, allow to release pressure naturally for 10 minutes then release remaining using quick release. Remove lid.
- ❖ Stir and serve.

Nutrition: Calories: 234;Fat: 4.8 g;Carbohydrates: 42.7 g;Sugar: 9 g;Protein: 7.3 g;Cholesterol: 0 mg

16) BANANA PEANUT BUTTER PUDDING

Cooking Time: 25 Minutes   **Servings: 1**

Ingredients:

- ✓ 2 bananas, halved
- ✓ ¼ cup smooth peanut butter
- ✓ Coconut for garnish, shredded

Directions:

- ❖ Start by blending bananas and peanut butter in a blender and mix until smooth or desired texture obtained.
- ❖ Pour into a bowl and garnish with coconut if desired.
- ❖ Enjoy.

Nutrition: Calories: 589, Total Fat: 33.3g, Saturated Fat: 6.9, Cholesterol: 0 mg, Sodium: 13 mg, Total Carbohydrate: 66.5 g, Dietary Fiber: 10 g, Total Sugars: 38 g, Protein: 18.8 g, Vitamin D: 0 mcg, Calcium: 40 mg, Iron: 2 mg, Potassium: 1264 mg

17) COCONUT BANANA MIX

Cooking Time: 4 Minutes   **Servings: 4**

Ingredients:

- ✓ 1 cup coconut milk
- ✓ 1 banana
- ✓ 1 cup dried coconut
- ✓ 2 tbsp ground flax seed
- ✓ 3 tbsp chopped raisins
- ✓ ⅛ tsp nutmeg
- ✓ ⅛ tsp cinnamon
- ✓ Salt to taste

Directions:

- ❖ Set a large skillet on the stove and set it to low heat.
- ❖ Chop up the banana.
- ❖ Pour the coconut milk, nutmeg, and cinnamon into the skillet.
- ❖ Pour in the ground flaxseed while stirring continuously.
- ❖ Add the dried coconut and banana. Mix the ingredients until combined well.
- ❖ Allow the mixture to simmer for 2 to 3 minutes while stirring occasionally.
- ❖ Set four airtight containers on the counter.
- ❖ Remove the pan from heat and sprinkle enough salt for your taste buds.
- ❖ Divide the mixture into the containers and place them into the fridge overnight. They can remain in the fridge for up to 3 days.
- ❖ Before you set this tasty mixture in the microwave to heat up, you need to let it thaw on the counter for a bit.

Nutrition: calories: 279, fats: 22 grams, carbohydrates: 25 grams, protein: 6.4 grams

18) OLIVE OIL RASPBERRY-LEMON MUFFINS

Cooking Time: 20 Minutes   **Servings: 12**

Ingredients:

- ✓ Cooking spray to grease baking liners
- ✓ 1 cup all-purpose flour
- ✓ 1 cup whole-wheat flour
- ✓ ½ cup tightly packed light brown sugar
- ✓ ½ tsp baking soda
- ✓ ½ tsp aluminum-free baking powder
- ✓ ⅛ tsp kosher salt
- ✓ 1¼ cups buttermilk
- ✓ 1 large egg
- ✓ ¼ cup extra-virgin olive oil
- ✓ 1 tbsp freshly squeezed lemon juice
- ✓ Zest of 2 lemons
- ✓ 1¼ cups frozen raspberries (do not thaw)

Directions:

- ❖ Preheat the oven to 400°F and line a muffin tin with baking liners. Spray the liners lightly with cooking spray.
- ❖ In a large mixing bowl, whisk together the all-purpose flour, whole-wheat flour, brown sugar, baking soda, baking powder, and salt.
- ❖ In a medium bowl, whisk together the buttermilk, egg, oil, lemon juice, and lemon zest.
- ❖ Pour the wet ingredients into the dry ingredients and stir just until blended. Do not overmix.
- ❖ Fold in the frozen raspberries.
- ❖ Scoop about ¼ cup of batter into each muffin liner and bake for 20 minutes, or until the tops look browned and a paring knife comes out clean when inserted. Remove the muffins from the tin to cool.
- ❖ STORAGE: Store covered containers at room temperature for up to 4 days. To freeze muffins for up to 3 months, wrap them in foil and place in an airtight resealable bag.

Nutrition: Total calories: 166; Total fat: 5g; Saturated fat: 1g; Sodium: 134mg; Carbohydrates: 30g; Fiber: 3g; Protein: 4g

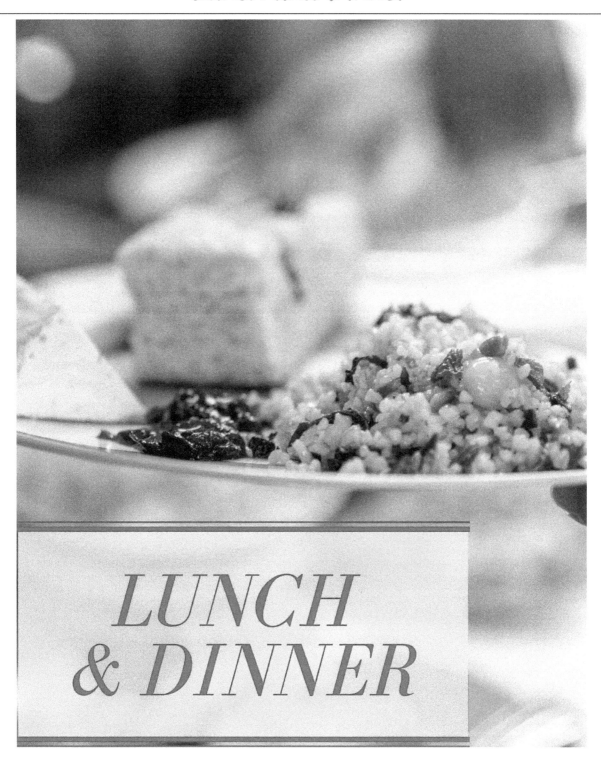

LUNCH
& DINNER

19) MARINATED TUNA STEAK SPECIAL

Cooking Time: 15-20 Minutes   **Servings:** 4

Ingredients:

- ✓ Olive oil (2 tbsp.)
- ✓ Orange juice (.25 cup)
- ✓ Soy sauce (.25 cup)
- ✓ Lemon juice (1 tbsp.)
- ✓ Fresh parsley (2 tbsp.)
- ✓ Garlic clove (1)
- ✓ Ground black pepper (.5 tsp.)
- ✓ Fresh oregano (.5 tsp.)
- ✓ Tuna steaks (4 - 4 oz. Steaks)

Directions:

- ❖ Mince the garlic and chop the oregano and parsley.
- ❖ In a glass container, mix the pepper, oregano, garlic, parsley, lemon juice, soy sauce, olive oil, and orange juice.
- ❖ Warm the grill using the high heat setting. Grease the grate with oil.
- ❖ Add to tuna steaks and cook for five to six minutes. Turn and baste with the marinated sauce.
- ❖ Cook another five minutes or until it's the way you like it. Discard the remaining marinade.

Nutrition: Calories: 200;Protein: 27.4 grams;Fat: 7.9 grams

20) SHRIMP AND GARLIC PASTA

Cooking Time: 15 Minutes   **Servings:** 4

Ingredients:

- ✓ 6 ounces whole wheat spaghetti
- ✓ 12 ounces raw shrimp, peeled and deveined, cut into 1-inch pieces
- ✓ 1 bunch asparagus, trimmed
- ✓ 1 large bell pepper, thinly sliced
- ✓ 1 cup fresh peas
- ✓ 3 garlic cloves, chopped
- ✓ 1 and ¼ tsp kosher salt
- ✓ ½ and ½ cups non-fat plain yogurt
- ✓ 3 tbsp lemon juice
- ✓ 1 tbsp extra-virgin olive oil
- ✓ ½ tsp fresh ground black pepper
- ✓ ¼ cup pine nuts, toasted

Directions:

- ❖ Take a large sized pot and bring water to a boil
- ❖ Add your spaghetti and cook them for about minutes less than the directed package instruction
- ❖ Add shrimp, bell pepper, asparagus and cook for about 2- 4 minutes until the shrimp are tender
- ❖ Drain the pasta and the contents well
- ❖ Take a large bowl and mash garlic until a paste form
- ❖ Whisk in yogurt, parsley, oil, pepper and lemon juice into the garlic paste
- ❖ Add pasta mix and toss well
- ❖ Serve by sprinkling some pine nuts!
- ❖ Enjoy!
- ❖ Meal Prep/Storage Options: Store in airtight containers in your fridge for 1-3 days.

Nutrition: Calories: 406;Fat: 22g;Carbohydrates: 28g;Protein: 26g

21) BUTTER PAPRIKA SHRIMPS

Cooking Time: 30 Minutes   **Servings:** 2

Ingredients:

- ✓ ¼ tbsp smoked paprika
- ✓ 1/8 cup sour cream
- ✓ ½ pound tiger shrimps
- ✓ 1/8 cup butter
- ✓ Salt and black pepper, to taste

Directions:

- ❖ Preheat the oven to 390 degrees F and grease a baking dish.
- ❖ Mix together all the ingredients in a large bowl and transfer into the baking dish.
- ❖ Place in the oven and bake for about 15 minutes.
- ❖ Place paprika shrimp in a dish and set aside to cool for meal prepping. Divide it in 2 containers and cover the lid. Refrigerate for 1-2 days and reheat in microwave before serving.

Nutrition: Calories: 330 ;Carbohydrates: 1.;Protein: 32.6g;Fat: 21.5g;Sugar: 0.2g;Sodium: 458mg

22) MEDITERRANEAN-STYLE SALMON AVOCADO SALAD

Cooking Time: 10 Minutes   **Servings:** 4

Ingredients:

- ✓ 1 lb skinless salmon fillets
- ✓ Marinade/Dressing:
- ✓ 3 tbsp olive oil
- ✓ 2 tbsp lemon juice fresh, squeezed
- ✓ 1 tbsp red wine vinegar, optional
- ✓ 1 tbsp fresh chopped parsley
- ✓ 2 tsp garlic minced
- ✓ Salad:
- ✓ 4 cups Romaine (or Cos) lettuce leaves, washed and dried
- ✓ 1 large cucumber, diced
- ✓ 2 Roma tomatoes, diced
- ✓ 1 red onion, sliced
- ✓ 1 avocado, sliced
- ✓ 1/2 cup feta cheese crumbled
- ✓ 1/3 cup pitted Kalamata olives or black olives, sliced

Directions:

- ❖ In a jug, whisk together the olive oil, lemon juice, red wine vinegar, chopped parsley, garlic minced, oregano, salt and pepper
- ❖ Pour out half of the marinade into a large, shallow dish, refrigerate the remaining marinade to use as the dressing
- ❖ Coat the salmon in the rest of the marinade
- ❖ Place a skillet pan or grill over medium-high, add 1 tbsp oil and sear

✓ 1 tsp dried oregano
✓ 1 tsp salt
✓ Cracked pepper, to taste

✓ Lemon wedges to serve

salmon on both sides until crispy and cooked through

❖ Allow the salmon to cool

❖ Distribute the salmon among the containers, store in the fridge for 2-3 days

❖ To Serve: Prepare the salad by placing the romaine lettuce, cucumber, roma tomatoes, red onion, avocado, feta cheese, and olives in a large salad bowl. Reheat the salmon in the microwave for 30seconds to 1 minute or until heated through.

❖ Slice the salmon and arrange over salad. Drizzle the salad with the remaining untouched dressing, serve with lemon wedges.

Nutrition: Calories:411;Carbs: 12g;Total Fat: 27g;Protein: 28g

23) KALE BEET SALAD

Cooking Time: 50 Minutes   **Servings: 6**

Ingredients:

✓ 1 bunch of kale, washed and dried, ribs removed, chopped
✓ 6 pieces washed beets, peeled and dried and cut into ½ inches
✓ ½ tsp dried rosemary
✓ ½ tsp garlic powder
✓ salt
✓ pepper
✓ olive oil
✓ ¼ medium red onion, thinly sliced

✓ 1-2 tbsp slivered almonds, toasted
✓ ¼ cup olive oil
✓ Juice of 1½ lemon
✓ ¼ cup honey
✓ ¼ tsp garlic powder
✓ 1 tsp dried rosemary
✓ salt
✓ pepper

Directions:

❖ Preheat oven to 400 degrees F.
❖ Take a bowl and toss the kale with some salt, pepper, and olive oil.
❖ Lightly oil a baking sheet and add the kale.
❖ Roast in the oven for 5 minutes, and then remove and place to the side.
❖ Place beets in a bowl and sprinkle with a bit of rosemary, garlic powder, pepper, and salt; ensure beets are coated well.
❖ Spread the beets on the oiled baking sheet, place on the middle rack of your oven, and roast for 45 minutes, turning twice.
❖ Make the lemon vinaigrette by whisking all of the listed Ingredients: in a bowl.
❖ Once the beets are ready, remove from the oven and allow it to cool.
❖ Take a medium-sized salad bowl and add kale, onions, and beets.
❖ Dress with lemon honey vinaigrette and toss well.
❖ Garnish with toasted almonds.
❖ Enjoy!

Nutrition: Calories: 245, Total Fat: 17.6 g, Saturated Fat: 2.6 g, Cholesterol: 0 mg, Sodium: 77 mg, Total Carbohydrate: 22.9 g, Dietary Fiber: 3 g, Total Sugars: 17.7 g, Protein: 2.4 g, Vitamin D: 0 mcg, Calcium: 50 mg, Iron: 1 mg, Potassium: 416 mg

24) MOROCCAN FISH

Cooking Time: 1 Hour 25 Minutes   **Servings:** 12

Ingredients:

- ✓ Garbanzo beans (15 oz. Can)
- ✓ Red bell peppers (2)
- ✓ Large carrot (1)
- ✓ Vegetable oil (1 tbsp.)
- ✓ Onion (1)
- ✓ Garlic (1 clove)
- ✓ Tomatoes (3 chopped/14.5 oz can)
- ✓ Olives (4 chopped)
- ✓ Chopped fresh parsley (.25 cup)
- ✓ Ground cumin (.25 cup)
- ✓ Paprika (3 tbsp.)
- ✓ Chicken bouillon granules (2 tbsp.)
- ✓ Cayenne pepper (1 tsp.)
- ✓ Salt (to your liking)
- ✓ Tilapia fillets (5 lb.)

Directions:

- ❖ Drain and rinse the beans. Thinly slice the carrot and onion. Mince the garlic and chop the olives. Discard the seeds from the peppers and slice them into strips.
- ❖ Warm the oil in a frying pan using the medium temperature setting. Toss in the onion and garlic. Simmer them for approximately five minutes.
- ❖ Fold in the bell peppers, beans, tomatoes, carrots, and olives.
- ❖ Continue sautéing them for about five additional minutes.
- ❖ Sprinkle the veggies with the cumin, parsley, salt, chicken bouillon, paprika, and cayenne.
- ❖ Stir thoroughly and place the fish on top of the veggies.
- ❖ Pour in water to cover the veggies.
- ❖ Lower the heat setting and cover the pan to slowly cook until the fish is flaky (about 40 min..

Nutrition: Calories: 268;Protein: 42 grams;Fat: 5 grams

25) SARDINES WITH NIÇOISE-INSPIRED SALAD

Cooking Time: 15 Minutes   **Servings:** 4

Ingredients:

- ✓ 4 eggs
- ✓ 12 ounces baby red potatoes (about 12 potatoes)
- ✓ 6 ounces green beans, halved
- ✓ 4 cups baby spinach leaves or mixed greens
- ✓ 1 bunch radishes, quartered (about 1⅓ cups)
- ✓ 1 cup cherry tomatoes
- ✓ 20 kalamata or niçoise olives (about ⅓ cup)
- ✓ 3 (3.75-ounce) cans skinless, boneless sardines packed in olive oil, drained
- ✓ 8 tbsp Dijon Red Wine Vinaigrette

Directions:

- ❖ Place the eggs in a saucepan and cover with water. Bring the water to a boil. As soon as the water starts to boil, place a lid on the pan and turn the heat off. Set a timer for minutes.
- ❖ When the timer goes off, drain the hot water and run cold water over the eggs to cool. Peel the eggs when cool and cut in half.
- ❖ Prick each potato a few times with a fork. Place them on a microwave-safe plate and microwave on high for 4 to 5 minutes, until the potatoes are tender. Let cool and cut in half.
- ❖ Place green beans on a microwave-safe plate and microwave on high for 1½ to 2 minutes, until the beans are crisp-tender. Cool.
- ❖ Place 1 egg, ½ cup of green beans, 6 potato halves, 1 cup of spinach, ⅓ cup of radishes, ¼ cup of tomatoes, olives, and 3 sardines in each of 4 containers. Pour 2 tbsp of vinaigrette into each of 4 sauce containers.
- ❖ STORAGE: Store covered containers in the refrigerator for up to 4 days.

Nutrition: Total calories: 450; Total fat: 32g; Saturated fat: 5g; Sodium: 6mg; Carbohydrates: 22g; Fiber: 5g; Protein: 21g

26) POMODORO LETTUCE SALAD

Cooking Time: 15 Minutes   **Servings:** 6

Ingredients:

- ✓ 1 heart of Romaine lettuce, chopped
- ✓ 3 Roma tomatoes, diced
- ✓ 1 English cucumber, diced
- ✓ 1 small red onion, finely chopped
- ✓ ½ cup curly parsley, finely chopped
- ✓ 2 tbsp virgin olive oil
- ✓ lemon juice, ½ large lemon
- ✓ 1 tsp garlic powder
- ✓ salt
- ✓ pepper

Directions:

- ❖ Add all Ingredients: to a large bowl.
- ❖ Toss well and transfer them to containers.
- ❖ Enjoy!

Nutrition: Calories: 68, Total Fat: 9 g, Saturated Fat: 0.8 g, Cholesterol: 0 mg, Sodium: 7 mg, Total Carbohydrate: 6 g, Dietary Fiber: 1.5 g, Total Sugars: 3.3 g, Protein: 1.3 g, Vitamin D: 0 mcg, Calcium: 18 mg, Iron: 1 mg, Potassium: 309 mg

27) MEDITERRANEAN-STYLE CHICKEN PASTA BAKE

Cooking Time: 30 Minutes   **Servings: 4**

Ingredients:

- ✓ Marinade:
- ✓ 1½ lbs. boneless, skinless chicken thighs, cut into bite-sized pieces*
- ✓ 2 garlic cloves, thinly sliced
- ✓ 2-3 tbsp. marinade from artichoke hearts
- ✓ 4 sprigs of fresh oregano, leaves stripped
- ✓ Olive oil
- ✓ Red wine vinegar
- ✓ Pasta:
- ✓ 1 lb whole wheat fusilli pasta
- ✓ 1 red onion, thinly sliced
- ✓ 1 pint grape or cherry tomatoes, whole
- ✓ ½ cup marinated artichoke hearts, roughly chopped
- ✓ ½ cup white beans, rinsed + drained (I use northern white beans)
- ✓ ½ cup Kalamata olives, roughly chopped
- ✓ ⅓ cup parsley and basil leaves, roughly chopped
- ✓ 2-3 handfuls of part-skim shredded mozzarella cheese
- ✓ Salt, to taste
- ✓ Pepper, to taste
- ✓ Garnish:
- ✓ Parsley
- ✓ Basil leaves

Directions:

- ❖ Create the chicken marinade by drain the artichoke hearts reserving the juice
- ❖ In a large bowl, add the artichoke juice, garlic, chicken, and oregano leaves, drizzle with olive oil, a splash of red wine vinegar, and mix well to coat
- ❖ Marinate for at least 1 hour, maximum hours
- ❖ Cook the pasta in boiling salted water, drain and set aside
- ❖ Preheat your oven to 42degrees F
- ❖ In a casserole dish, add the sliced onions and tomatoes, toss with olive oil, salt and pepper. Then cook, stirring occasionally, until the onions are soft and the tomatoes start to burst, about 15-20 minutes
- ❖ In the meantime, in a large skillet over medium heat, add 1 tsp of olive oil
- ❖ Remove the chicken from the marinade, pat dry, and season with salt and pepper
- ❖ Working in batches, brown the chicken on both sides, leaving slightly undercooked
- ❖ Remove the casserole dish from the oven, add in the cooked pasta, browned chicken, artichoke hearts, beans, olives, and chopped herbs, stir to combine
- ❖ Top with grated cheese
- ❖ Bake for an additional 5-7 minutes, until the cheese is brown and bubbling
- ❖ Remove from the oven and allow the dish to cool completely
- ❖ Distribute among the containers, store for 2-3 days
- ❖ To Serve: Reheat in the microwave for 1-2 minutes or until heated through.
- ❖ Garnish with fresh herbs and serve

Nutrition: Calories:487;Carbs: 95g;Total Fat: 5g;Protein: 22g

28) VEGETABLE FLATBREAD ROAST

Cooking Time: 25 Minutes   **Servings: 12**

Ingredients:

- ✓ 16 oz pizza dough, homemade or frozen
- ✓ 6 oz soft goat cheese, divided
- ✓ ¾ cup grated Parmesan cheese divided
- ✓ 3 tbsp chopped fresh dill, divided
- ✓ 1 small red onion, sliced thinly
- ✓ 1 small zucchini, sliced thinly
- ✓ 2 small tomatoes, thinly sliced
- ✓ 1 small red pepper, thinly sliced into rings
- ✓ Olive oil
- ✓ Salt, to taste
- ✓ Pepper, to taste

Directions:

- ❖ Preheat the oven to 400 degrees F
- ❖ Roll the dough into a large rectangle, and then place it on a piece of parchment paper sprayed with non-stick spray
- ❖ Take a knife and spread half the goat cheese onto one half of the dough, then sprinkle with half the dill and half the Parmesan cheese
- ❖ Carefully fold the other half of the dough on top of the cheese, spread and sprinkle the remaining parmesan and goat cheese
- ❖ Layer the thinly sliced vegetables over the top
- ❖ Brush the olive oil over the top of the veggies and sprinkle with salt, pepper, and the remaining dill
- ❖ Bake for 22-25 minutes, until the edges are medium brown, cut in half, lengthwise
- ❖ Then slice the flatbread in long 2-inch slices and allow to cool
- ❖ Distribute among the containers, store for 2 days
- ❖ To Serve: Reheat in the oven at 375 degrees for 5 minutes or until hot. Enjoy with a fresh salad.

Nutrition: Calories:170;Carbs: 21g;Total Fat: 6g;Protein: 8g

29) COBB SALAD WITH STEAK

Cooking Time: 15 Minutes   **Servings: 4**

Ingredients:

- ✓ 6 large eggs
- ✓ 2 tbsp unsalted butter
- ✓ 1 lb steak
- ✓ 2 tbsp olive oil
- ✓ 6 cups baby spinach

- ✓ 1 cup cherry tomatoes, halved
- ✓ 1 cup pecan halves
- ✓ 1/2 cup crumbled feta cheese
- ✓ Kosher salt, to taste
- ✓ Freshly ground black pepper, to taste

Directions:

- ❖ In a large skillet over medium high heat, melt butter
- ❖ Using paper towels, pat the steak dry, then drizzle with olive oil and season with salt and pepper, to taste
- ❖ Once heated, add the steak to the skillet and cook, flipping once, until cooked through to desired doneness, - cook for 4 minutes per side for a medium-rare steak
- ❖ Transfer the steak to a plate and allow it to cool before dicing
- ❖ Place the eggs in a large saucepan and cover with cold water by 1 inch
- ❖ Bring to a boil and cook for 1 minute, cover the eggs with a tight-fitting lid and remove from heat, set aside for 8-10 minutes, then drain well and allow to cool before peeling and dicing
- ❖ Assemble the salad in the container by placing the spinach at the bottom of the container, top with arranged rows of steak, eggs, feta, tomatoes, and pecans
- ❖ To Serve: Top with the balsamic vinaigrette, or desired dressing
- ❖ Recipe Note: You can also use New York, rib-eye or filet mignon for this recipe

Nutrition: Calories:640;Total Fat: 51g;Total Carbs: 9.8g;Fiber: 5g;Protein: 38.8g

30) LAMB CHOPS GRILL

Cooking Time: 10 Minutes   **Servings: 4**

Ingredients:

- ✓ 4 8-ounce lamb shoulder chops
- ✓ 2 tbsp Dijon mustard
- ✓ 2 tbsp balsamic vinegar

- ✓ 1 tbsp chopped garlic
- ✓ ¼ tsp ground black pepper
- ✓ ½ cup olive oil
- ✓ 2 tbsp fresh basil, shredded

Directions:

- ❖ Pat the lamb chops dry and arrange them in a shallow glass-baking dish.
- ❖ Take a bowl and whisk in Dijon mustard, garlic, balsamic vinegar, and pepper.
- ❖ Mix well to make the marinade.
- ❖ Whisk oil slowly into the marinade until it is smooth.
- ❖ Stir in basil.
- ❖ Pour the marinade over the lamb chops, making sure to coat both sides.
- ❖ Cover, refrigerate and allow the chops to marinate for anywhere from 1-4 hours.
- ❖ Remove the chops from the refrigerator and leave out for 30 minutes or until room temperature.
- ❖ Preheat grill to medium heat and oil grate.
- ❖ Grill the lamb chops until the center reads 145 degrees F and they are nicely browned, about 5-minutes per side.
- ❖ Enjoy!

Nutrition: Calories: 1587, Total Fat: 97.5 g, Saturated Fat: 27.6 g, Cholesterol: 600 mg, Sodium: 729 mg, Total Carbohydrate: 1.3 g, Dietary Fiber: 0.4 g, Total Sugars: 0.1 g, Protein: 176.5 g, Vitamin D: 0 mcg, Calcium: 172 mg, Iron: 15 mg, Potassium: 30 mg

31) CHILI BROILED CALAMARI

Cooking Time: 8 Minutes   **Servings: 4**

Ingredients:

- 2 tbsp extra virgin olive oil
- 1 tsp chili powder
- ½ tsp ground cumin
- Zest of 1 lime
- Juice of 1 lime
- Dash of sea salt
- 1 and ½ pounds squid, cleaned and split open, with tentacles cut into ½ inch rounds
- 2 tbsp cilantro, chopped
- 2 tbsp red bell pepper, minced

Directions:

- Take a medium bowl and stir in olive oil, chili powder, cumin, lime zest, sea salt, lime juice and pepper
- Add squid and let it marinade and stir to coat, coat and let it refrigerate for 1 hour
- Pre-heat your oven to broil
- Arrange squid on a baking sheet, broil for 8 minutes turn once until tender
- Garnish the broiled calamari with cilantro and red bell pepper
- Serve and enjoy!
- Meal Prep/Storage Options: Store in airtight containers in your fridge for 1-2 days.

Nutrition: Calories:159;Fat: 13g;Carbohydrates: 12g;Protein: 3g

32) SALMON AND CORN PEPPER SALSA

Cooking Time: 12 Minutes   **Servings: 2**

Ingredients:

- 1 garlic clove, grated
- ½ tsp mild chili powder
- ½ tsp ground coriander
- ¼ tsp ground cumin
- 2 limes – 1, zest and juice; 1 cut into wedges
- 2 tsp rapeseed oil
- 2 wild salmon fillets
- 1 ear of corn on the cob, husk removed
- 1 red onion, finely chopped
- 1 avocado, cored, peeled, and finely chopped
- 1 red pepper, deseeded and finely chopped
- 1 red chili, halved and deseeded
- ½ a pack of finely chopped coriander

Directions:

- Boil the corn in water for about 6-8 minutes until tender.
- Drain and cut off the kernels.
- In a bowl, combine garlic, spices, 1 tbsp of limejuice, and oil; mix well to prepare spice rub.
- Coat the salmon with the rub.
- Add the zest to the corn and give it a gentle stir.
- Heat a frying pan over medium heat.
- Add salmon and cook for about 2 minutes per side.
- Serve the cooked salmon with salsa and lime wedges.
- Enjoy!

Nutrition: Calories: 949, Total Fat: 57.4 g, Saturated Fat: 9.7 g, Cholesterol: 2mg, Sodium: 180 mg, Total Carbohydrate: 33.5 g, Dietary Fiber: 11.8 g, Total Sugars: 8.3 g, Protein: 76.8 g, Vitamin D: 0 mcg, Calcium: 100 mg, Iron: 3 mg, Potassium: 856 mg

33) ITALIAN-INSPIRED ROTISSERIE CHICKEN WITH BROCCOLI SLAW

Cooking Time: 15 Minutes   **Servings: 4**

Ingredients:

- 4 cups packaged broccoli slaw
- 1 cooked rotisserie chicken, meat removed (about 10 to 12 ounces)
- 1 bunch red radishes, stemmed, halved, and thickly sliced (about 1¼ cups)
- 1 cup sliced red onion
- ½ cup pitted kalamata or niçoise olives, roughly chopped
- ½ cup sliced pepperoncini
- 8 tbsp Dijon Red Wine Vinaigrette, divided

Directions:

- Place the broccoli slaw, chicken, radishes, onion, olives, and pepperoncini in a large mixing bowl. Toss to combine.
- Place cups of salad in each of 4 containers. Pour 2 tbsp of vinaigrette into each of 4 sauce containers.
- STORAGE: Store covered containers in the refrigerator for up to 5 days.

Nutrition: Total calories: 329; Total fat: 2; Saturated fat: 4g; Sodium: 849mg; Carbohydrates: 10g; Fiber: 3g; Protein: 20g

34) FLATBREAD AND ROASTED VEGETABLES

Cooking Time: 45 Minutes   **Servings: 12**

Ingredients:

- ✓ 5 ounces goat cheese
- ✓ 1 thinly sliced onion
- ✓ 2 thinly sliced tomatoes
- ✓ Olive oil
- ✓ ¼ tsp pepper
- ✓ ⅛ tsp salt
- ✓ 16 ounces homemade or frozen pizza dough
- ✓ ¾ tbsp chopped dill, fresh is better
- ✓ 1 thinly sliced zucchini
- ✓ 1 red pepper, cup into rings

Directions:

- ❖ Set your oven to 400 degrees Fahrenheit.
- ❖ Set the dough on a large piece of parchment paper. Use a rolling pin to roll the dough into a large rectangle.
- ❖ Spread half of the goat cheese on ½ of the pizza dough.
- ❖ Sprinkle half of the dill on the other half of the dough.
- ❖ Fold the dough so the half with the dill is on top of the cheese.
- ❖ Spread the remaining goat cheese on the pizza dough and then sprinkle the rest of the dill over the cheese.
- ❖ Layer the vegetables on top in any arrangement you like.
- ❖ Drizzle olive oil on top of the vegetables.
- ❖ Sprinkle salt and pepper over the olive oil.
- ❖ Set the piece of parchment paper on a pizza pan or baking pan and place it in the oven.
- ❖ Set the timer for 22 minutes. If the edges are not a medium brown, leave the flatbread in the oven for another couple of minutes.
- ❖ Remove the pizza from the oven when it is done and cut the flatbread in half lengthwise.
- ❖ Slice the flatbread into 2-inch long pieces and enjoy!

Nutrition: calories: 170, fats: 5 grams, carbohydrates: 20 grams, protein: 8 grams.

35) SEAFOOD RICE

Cooking Time: 40 Minutes   **Servings: 4-5**

Ingredients:

- ✓ 4 small lobster tails (6-12 oz each)
- ✓ Water
- ✓ 3 tbsp Extra Virgin Olive Oil
- ✓ 1 large yellow onion, chopped
- ✓ 2 cups Spanish rice or short grain rice, soaked in water for 15 minutes and then drained
- ✓ 4 garlic cloves, chopped
- ✓ 2 large pinches of Spanish saffron threads soaked in 1/2 cup water
- ✓ 1 tsp Sweet Spanish paprika
- ✓ 1 tsp cayenne pepper
- ✓ 1/2 tsp aleppo pepper flakes
- ✓ Salt, to taste
- ✓ 2 large Roma tomatoes, finely chopped
- ✓ 6 oz French green beans, trimmed
- ✓ 1 lb prawns or large shrimp or your choice, peeled and deveined
- ✓ 1/4 cup chopped fresh parsley

Directions:

- ❖ In a large pot, add 3 cups of water and bring it to a rolling boil
- ❖ Add in the lobster tails and allow boil briefly, about 1-minutes or until pink, remove from heat
- ❖ Using tongs transfer the lobster tails to a plate and Do not discard the lobster cooking water
- ❖ Allow the lobster is cool, then remove the shell and cut into large chunks.
- ❖ In a large deep pan or skillet over medium-high heat, add 3 tbsp olive oil
- ❖ Add the chopped onions, sauté the onions for 2 minutes and then add the rice, and cook for 3 more minutes, stirring regularly
- ❖ Then add in the lobster cooking water and the chopped garlic and, stir in the saffron and its soaking liquid, cayenne pepper, aleppo pepper, paprika, and salt
- ❖ Gently stir in the chopped tomatoes and green beans, bring to a boil and allow the liquid slightly reduce, then cover (with lid or tightly wrapped foil) and cook over low heat for 20 minutes
- ❖ Once done, uncover and spread the shrimp over the rice, push it into the rice slightly, add in a little water, if needed
- ❖ Cover and cook for another 15 minutes until the shrimp turn pink
- ❖ Then add in the cooked lobster chunks
- ❖ Once the lobster is warmed through, remove from heat allow the dish to cool completely
- ❖ Distribute among the containers, store for 2 days
- ❖ To Serve: Reheat in the microwave for 1-2 minutes or until heated through. Garnish with parsley and enjoy!
- ❖ Recipe Notes: Remember to soak your rice if needed to help with the cooking process

Nutrition: Calories:536;Carbs: 56g;Total Fat: 26g;Protein: 50g

Soups and Salads Recipes

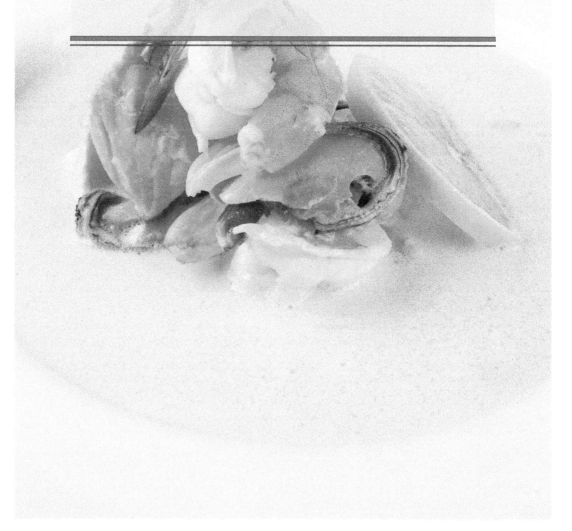

SOUPS & SALADS

36) MEXICAN-STYLE TORTILLA SOUP

Cooking Time: 40 Minutes   **Servings:** 4

Ingredients:

- ✓ 1-pound chicken breasts, boneless and skinless
- ✓ 1 can (15 ounces whole peeled tomatoes
- ✓ 1 can (10 ounces red enchilada sauce
- ✓ 1 and 1/2 tsp minced garlic
- ✓ 1 yellow onion, diced
- ✓ 1 can (4 ounces fire-roasted diced green chile
- ✓ 1 can (15 ounces black beans, drained and rinsed

- ✓ 1 can (15 ounces fire-roasted corn, undrained
- ✓ 1 container (32 ounces chicken stock or broth
- ✓ 1 tsp ground cumin
- ✓ 2 tsp chili powder
- ✓ 3/4 tsp paprika
- ✓ 1 bay leaf
- ✓ Salt and freshly cracked pepper, to taste
- ✓ 1 tbsp chopped cilantro
- ✓ Tortilla strips, Freshly squeezed lime juice, freshly grated cheddar cheese,

Directions:

- ❖ Set your Instant Pot on Sauté mode.
- ❖ Toss olive oil, onion and garlic into the insert of the Instant Pot.
- ❖ Sauté for 4 minutes then add chicken and remaining ingredients.
- ❖ Mix well gently then seal and lock the lid.
- ❖ Select Manual mode for 7 minutes at high pressure.
- ❖ Once done, release the pressure completely then remove the lid.
- ❖ Adjust seasoning as needed.
- ❖ Garnish with desired toppings.
- ❖ Enjoy.

Nutrition: Calories: 390;Carbohydrate: 5.6g;Protein: 29.5g;Fat: 26.5g;Sugar: 2.1g;Sodium: 620mg

37) MEDITERRANEAN CHICKEN NOODLE SOUP

Cooking Time: 35 Minutes   **Servings:** 6

Ingredients:

- ✓ 1 tbsp olive oil
- ✓ 1 1/2 cups peeled and diced carrots
- ✓ 1 1/2 cup diced celery
- ✓ 1 cup chopped yellow onion
- ✓ 3 tbsp minced garlic
- ✓ 8 cups low-sodium chicken broth
- ✓ 2 tsp minced fresh thyme

- ✓ 2 tsp minced fresh rosemary
- ✓ 1 bay leaf
- ✓ salt and freshly ground black pepper
- ✓ 2 1/2 lbs. bone-in, skin-on chicken thighs, skinned
- ✓ 3 cups wide egg noodles, such as American beauty
- ✓ 1 tbsp fresh lemon juice
- ✓ 1/4 cup chopped fresh parsley

Directions:

- ❖ Preheat olive oil in the insert of the Instant Pot on Sauté mode.
- ❖ Add onion, celery, and carrots and sauté them for minutes.
- ❖ Stir in garlic and sauté for 1 minute.
- ❖ Add bay leaf, thyme, broth, rosemary, salt, and pepper.
- ❖ Seal and secure the Instant Pot lid and select Manual mode for 10 minutes at high pressure.
- ❖ Once done, release the pressure completely then remove the lid.
- ❖ Add noodles to the insert and switch the Instant Pot to sauté mode.
- ❖ Cook the soup for 6 minutes until noodles are all done.
- ❖ Remove the chicken and shred it using a fork.
- ❖ Return the chicken to the soup then add lemon juice and parsley.
- ❖ Enjoy.

Nutrition: Calories: 333;Carbohydrate: 3.3g;Protein: 44.7g;Fat: 13.7g;Sugar: 1.1g;Sodium: 509mg

38) SPECIAL TURKEY ARUGULA SALAD

Cooking Time: 5 Minutes   **Servings:** 2

Ingredients:

- ✓ 4 oz turkey breast meat, diced into small pieces
- ✓ 3.5 oz arugula leaves

- ✓ 10 raspberries
- ✓ Juice from ½ a lime
- ✓ 2 tbsp extra virgin olive oil

Directions:

- ❖ Mix together the turkey with the rest of the ingredients in a large bowl until well combined.
- ❖ Dish out in a glass bowl and serve immediately.

Nutrition: Calories: 246;Carbs: 15.4g;Fats: 15.9g;Proteins: 12.2g;Sodium: 590mg;Sugar: 7.6g

39) SPECIAL CHEESY BROCCOLI SOUP

Cooking Time: 30 Minutes   **Servings: 4**

Ingredients:

- ½ cup heavy whipping cream
- 1 cup broccoli
- ✓ 1 cup cheddar cheese
- ✓ Salt, to taste
- ✓ 1½ cups chicken broth

Directions:

- ❖ Heat chicken broth in a large pot and add broccoli.
- ❖ Bring to a boil and stir in the rest of the ingredients.
- ❖ Allow the soup to simmer on low heat for about 20 minutes.
- ❖ Ladle out into a bowl and serve hot.

Nutrition: Calories: 188;Carbs: 2.6g;Fats: 15g;Proteins: 9.8g;Sodium: 514mg;Sugar: 0.8g

40) DELICIOUS RICH POTATO SOUP

Cooking Time: 30 Minutes   **Servings: 4**

Ingredients:

- 1 tbsp butter
- 1 medium onion, diced
- 3 cloves garlic, minced
- 3 cups chicken broth
- 1 can/box cream of chicken soup
- 7-8 medium-sized russet potatoes, peeled and chopped
- 1 1/2 tsp salt
- ✓ Black pepper to taste
- ✓ 1 cup milk
- ✓ 1 tbsp flour
- ✓ 2 cups shredded cheddar cheese
- ✓ Garnish:
- ✓ 5-6 slices bacon, chopped
- ✓ Sliced green onions
- ✓ Shredded cheddar cheese

Directions:

- ❖ Heat butter in the insert of the Instant Pot on sauté mode.
- ❖ Add onions and sauté for 4 minutes until soft.
- ❖ Stir in garlic and sauté it for 1 minute.
- ❖ Add potatoes, cream of chicken, broth, salt, and pepper to the insert.
- ❖ Mix well then seal and lock the lid.
- ❖ Cook this mixture for 10 minutes at Manual Mode with high pressure.
- ❖ Meanwhile, mix flour with milk in a bowl and set it aside.
- ❖ Once the instant pot beeps, release the pressure completely.
- ❖ Remove the Instant Pot lid and switch the instant pot to Sauté mode.
- ❖ Pour in flour slurry and stir cook the mixture for 5 minutes until it thickens.
- ❖ Add 2 cups of cheddar cheese and let it melt.
- ❖ Garnish it as desired.
- ❖ Serve.

Nutrition: Calories: 784;Carbohydrate: 54.8g;Protein: 34g;Fat: 46.5g;Sugar: 7.5g;Sodium: 849mg

41) MEDITERRANEAN-STYLE LENTIL SOUP

Cooking Time: 20 Minutes   **Servings: 4**

Ingredients:

- 1 tbsp olive oil
- 1/2 cup red lentils
- 1 medium yellow or red onion
- 2 garlic cloves, chopped
- 1/2 tsp ground cumin
- 1/2 tsp ground coriander
- ✓ 1/2 tsp ground sumac
- ✓ 1/2 tsp red chili flakes
- ✓ 1/2 tsp dried parsley
- ✓ 3/4 tsp dried mint flakes
- ✓ pinch of sugar
- ✓ 2.5 cups water
- ✓ salt, to taste
- ✓ black pepper, to taste
- ✓ juice of 1/2 lime
- ✓ parsley or cilantro, to garnish

Directions:

- ❖ Preheat oil in the insert of your Instant Pot on Sauté mode.
- ❖ Add onion and sauté until it turns golden brown.
- ❖ Toss in the garlic, parsley sugar, mint flakes, red chili flakes, sumac, coriander, and cumin.
- ❖ Stir cook this mixture for 2 minutes.
- ❖ Add water, lentils, salt, and pepper. Stir gently.
- ❖ Seal and lock the Instant Pot lid and select Manual mode for 8 minutes at high pressure.
- ❖ Once done, release the pressure completely then remove the lid.
- ❖ Stir well then add lime juice.
- ❖ Serve warm.

Nutrition: Calories: 525;Carbohydrate: 59.8g;Protein: 30.1g;Fat: 19.3g;Sugar: 17.3g;Sodium: 897mg

42) DELICIOUS CREAMY KETO CUCUMBER SALAD

Cooking Time: 5 Minutes   **Servings:** 2

Ingredients:

- 2 tbsp mayonnaise
- Salt and black pepper, to taste
- 1 cucumber, sliced and quartered
- 2 tbsp lemon juice

Directions:

- Mix together the mayonnaise, cucumber slices, and lemon juice in a large bowl.
- Season with salt and black pepper and combine well.
- Dish out in a glass bowl and serve while it is cold.

Nutrition: Calories: 8Carbs: 9.3g;Fats: 5.2g;Proteins: 1.2g;Sodium: 111mg;Sugar: 3.8g

43) SAUSAGE KALE SOUP AND MUSHROOMS

Cooking Time: 1 Hour 10 Minutes   **Servings:** 6

Ingredients:

- 2 cups fresh kale, cut into bite sized pieces
- 6.5 ounces mushrooms, sliced
- 6 cups chicken bone broth
- 1 pound sausage, cooked and sliced
- Salt and black pepper, to taste

Directions:

- Heat chicken broth with two cans of water in a large pot and bring to a boil.
- Stir in the rest of the ingredients and allow the soup to simmer on low heat for about 1 hour.
- Dish out and serve hot.

Nutrition: Calories: 259;Carbs: ;Fats: 20g;Proteins: 14g;Sodium: 995mg;Sugar: 0.6g

44) CLASSIC MINESTRONE SOUP

Cooking Time: 25 Minutes   **Servings:** 6

Ingredients:

- 2 tbsp olive oil
- 3 cloves garlic, minced
- 1 onion, diced
- 2 carrots, peeled and diced
- 2 stalks celery, diced
- 1 1/2 tsp dried basil
- 1 tsp dried oregano
- 1/2 tsp fennel seed
- 6 cups low sodium chicken broth
- 1 (28-ounce can diced tomatoes
- 1 (16-ounce can kidney beans, drained and rinsed
- 1 zucchini, chopped
- 1 (3-inch Parmesan rind
- 1 bay leaf
- 1 bunch kale leaves, chopped
- 2 tsp red wine vinegar
- Kosher salt and black pepper, to taste
- 1/3 cup freshly grated Parmesan
- 2 tbsp chopped fresh parsley leaves

Directions:

- Preheat olive oil in the insert of the Instant Pot on Sauté mode.
- Add carrots, celery, and onion, sauté for 3 minutes.
- Stir in fennel seeds, oregano, and basil. Stir cook for 1 minute.
- Add stock, beans, tomatoes, parmesan, bay leaf, and zucchini.
- Secure and seal the Instant Pot lid then select Manual mode to cook for minutes at high pressure.
- Once done, release the pressure completely then remove the lid.
- Add kale and let it sit for 2 minutes in the hot soup.
- Stir in red wine, vinegar, pepper, and salt.
- Garnish with parsley and parmesan.
- Enjoy.

Nutrition: Calories: 805;Carbohydrate: 2.5g;Protein: 124.1g;Fat: 34g;Sugar: 1.4g;Sodium: 634mg

45) SPECIAL KOMBU SEAWEED SALAD

Cooking Time: 40 Minutes   **Servings:** 6

Ingredients:

- 4 garlic cloves, crushed
- 1 pound fresh kombu seaweed, boiled and cut into strips
- 2 tbsp apple cider vinegar
- Salt, to taste
- 2 tbsp coconut aminos

Directions:

- Mix together the kombu, garlic, apple cider vinegar, and coconut aminos in a large bowl.
- Season with salt and combine well.
- Dish out in a glass bowl and serve immediately.

Nutrition: Calories: 257;Carbs: 16.9g;Fats: 19.;Proteins: 6.5g;Sodium: 294mg;Sugar: 2.7g

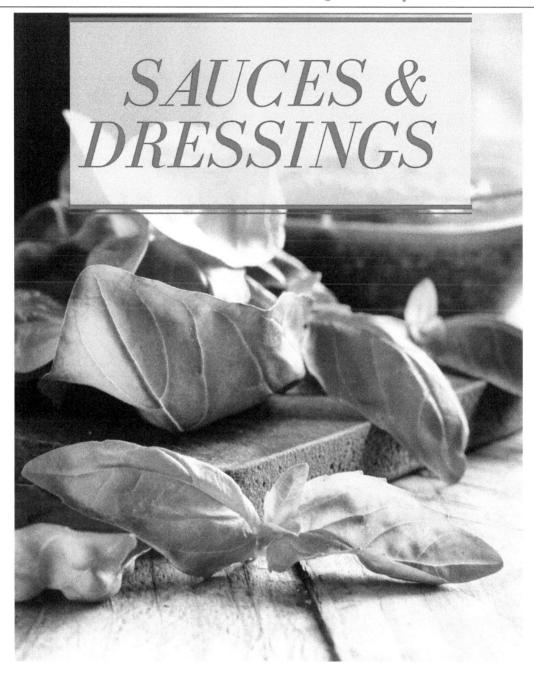

46) SPECIAL POMEGRANATE VINAIGRETTE

Cooking Time: 5 Minutes **Servings:** ½ Cup

Ingredients:

- ⅓ cup pomegranate juice
- 1 tsp Dijon mustard
- 1 tbsp apple cider vinegar
- ½ tsp dried mint
- 2 tbsp plus 2 tsp olive oil

Directions:

- ❖ Place the pomegranate juice, mustard, vinegar, and mint in a small bowl and whisk to combine.
- ❖ Whisk in the oil, pouring it into the bowl in a thin steam.
- ❖ Pour the vinaigrette into a container and refrigerate.
- ❖ STORAGE: Store the covered container in the refrigerator for up to 2 weeks. Bring the vinaigrette to room temperature and shake before serving.

Nutrition: (2 tbsp): Total calories: 94; Total fat: 10g; Saturated fat: 2g; Sodium: 30mg; Carbohydrates: 3g; Fiber: 0g; Protein: 0g

47) GREEN OLIVE WITH SPINACH TAPENADE

Cooking Time: 20 Minutes **Servings:** 1½ Cups

Ingredients:

- 1 cup pimento-stuffed green olives, drained
- 3 packed cups baby spinach
- 1 tsp chopped garlic
- ½ tsp dried oregano
- ⅓ cup packed fresh basil
- 2 tbsp olive oil
- 2 tsp red wine vinegar

Directions:

- ❖ Place all the ingredients in the bowl of a food processor and pulse until the mixture looks finely chopped but not puréed.
- ❖ Scoop the tapenade into a container and refrigerate.
- ❖ STORAGE: Store the covered container in the refrigerator for up to 5 days.

Nutrition: (¼ cup): Total calories: 80; Total fat: 8g; Saturated fat: 1g; Sodium: 6mg; Carbohydrates: 1g; Fiber: 1g; Protein: 1g

48) BULGUR PILAF AND ALMONDS

Cooking Time: 20 Minutes **Servings:** 4

Ingredients:

- ⅔ cup uncooked bulgur
- 1⅓ cups water
- ¼ cup sliced almonds
- 1 cup small diced red bell pepper
- ⅓ cup chopped fresh cilantro
- 1 tbsp olive oil
- ¼ tsp salt

Directions:

- ❖ Place the bulgur and water in a saucepan and bring the water to a boil. Once the water is at a boil, cover the pot with a lid and turn off the heat. Let the covered pot stand for 20 minutes.
- ❖ Transfer the cooked bulgur to a large mixing bowl and add the almonds, peppers, cilantro, oil, and salt. Stir to combine.
- ❖ Place about 1 cup of bulgur in each of 4 containers.
- ❖ STORAGE: Store covered containers in the refrigerator for up to 5 days. Bulgur can be either reheated or eaten at room temperature.

Nutrition: Total calories: 17 Total fat: 7g; Saturated fat: 1g; Sodium: 152mg; Carbohydrates: 25g; Fiber: 6g; Protein: 4g

49) SPANISH GARLIC YOGURT SAUCE

Cooking Time: 5 Minutes **Servings:** 1 Cup

Ingredients:

- 1 cup low-fat (2%) plain Greek yogurt
- ½ tsp garlic powder
- 1 tbsp freshly squeezed lemon juice
- 1 tbsp olive oil
- ¼ tsp kosher salt

Directions:

- ❖ Mix all the ingredients in a medium bowl until well combined.
- ❖ Spoon the yogurt sauce into a container and refrigerate.
- ❖ STORAGE: Store the covered container in the refrigerator for up to 7 days

Nutrition: (¼ cup): Total calories: 75; Total fat: 5g; Saturated fat: 1g; Sodium: 173mg; Carbohydrates: 3g; Fiber: 0g; Protein: 6g.

50) ORANGE WITH CINNAMON–SCENTED WHOLE-WHEAT COUSCOUS

Cooking Time: 10 Minutes   **Servings: 4**

Ingredients:

- ✓ 2 tsp olive oil
- ✓ ¼ cup minced shallot
- ✓ ½ cup freshly squeezed orange juice (from 2 oranges)
- ✓ ½ cup water
- ✓ ⅛ tsp ground cinnamon
- ✓ ¼ tsp kosher salt
- ✓ 1 cup whole-wheat couscous

Directions:

- ❖ Heat the oil in a saucepan over medium heat. Once the oil is shimmering, add the shallot and cook for 2 minutes, stirring frequently. Add the orange juice, water, cinnamon, and salt, and bring to a boil.
- ❖ Once the liquid is boiling, add the couscous, cover the pan, and turn off the heat. Leave the couscous covered for 5 minutes. When the couscous is done, fluff with a fork.
- ❖ Place ¾ cup of couscous in each of 4 containers.
- ❖ STORAGE: Store covered containers in the refrigerator for up to 5 days. Freeze for up to 2 months.

Nutrition: Total calories: 21 Total fat: 4g; Saturated fat: <1g; Sodium: 147mg; Carbohydrates: 41g; Fiber: 5g; Protein: 8g

51) CHUNKY ROASTED CHERRY TOMATO WITH BASIL SAUCE

Cooking Time: 40 Minutes   **Servings: 1⅓ Cups**

Ingredients:

- ✓ 2 pints cherry tomatoes (20 ounces total)
- ✓ 2 tsp olive oil, plus 3 tbsp
- ✓ ¼ tsp kosher salt
- ✓ ½ tsp chopped garlic
- ✓ ¼ cup fresh basil leaves

Directions:

- ❖ Preheat the oven to 350°F. Line a sheet pan with a silicone baking mat or parchment paper.
- ❖ Place the tomatoes on the lined sheet pan and toss with tsp of oil. Roast for 40 minutes, shaking the pan halfway through.
- ❖ While the tomatoes are still warm, place them in a medium mixing bowl and add the salt, the garlic, and the remaining tbsp of oil. Mash the tomatoes with the back of a fork. Stir in the fresh basil.
- ❖ Scoop the sauce into a container and refrigerate.
- ❖ STORAGE: Store the covered container in the refrigerator for up to days.

Nutrition: (⅓ cup): Total calories: 141; Total fat: 13g; Saturated fat: 2g; Sodium: 158mg; Carbohydrates: 7g; Fiber: 2g; Protein: 1g

52) CELERY HEART, BASIL, AND ALMOND PESTO

Cooking Time: 10 Minutes   **Servings: 1 Cup**

Ingredients:

- ✓ ½ cup raw, unsalted almonds
- ✓ 3 cups fresh basil leaves, (about 1½ ounces)
- ✓ ½ cup chopped celery hearts with leaves
- ✓ ¼ tsp kosher salt
- ✓ 1 tbsp freshly squeezed lemon juice
- ✓ ¼ cup olive oil
- ✓ 3 tbsp water

Directions:

- ❖ Place the almonds in the bowl of a food processor and process until they look like coarse sand.
- ❖ Add the basil, celery hearts, salt, lemon juice, oil and water and process until smooth. The sauce will be somewhat thick. If you would like a thinner sauce, add more water, oil, or lemon juice, depending on your taste preference.
- ❖ Scoop the pesto into a container and refrigerate.
- ❖ STORAGE: Store the covered container in the refrigerator for up to 2 weeks. Pesto may be frozen for up to 6 months.

Nutrition: (¼ cup): Total calories: 231; Total fat: 22g; Saturated fat: 3g; Sodium: 178mg; Carbohydrates: 6g; Fiber: 3g; Protein: 4g

53) SAUTÉED KALE AND GARLIC WITH LEMON

Cooking Time: 7 Minutes   **Servings: 4**

Ingredients:

- ✓ 1 tbsp olive oil
- ✓ 3 bunches kale, stemmed and roughly chopped
- ✓ 2 tsp chopped garlic
- ✓ ¼ tsp kosher salt
- ✓ 1 tbsp freshly squeezed lemon juice

Directions:

- ❖ Heat the oil in a -inch skillet over medium-high heat. Once the oil is shimmering, add as much kale as will fit in the pan. You will probably only fit half the leaves into the pan at first. Mix the kale with tongs so that the leaves are coated with oil and start to wilt. As the kale wilts, keep adding more of the raw kale, continuing to use tongs to mix. Once all the kale is in the pan, add the garlic and salt and continue to cook until the kale is tender. Total cooking time from start to finish should be about 7 minutes.
- ❖ Mix the lemon juice into the kale. Add additional salt and/or lemon juice if necessary. Place 1 cup of kale in each of 4 containers and refrigerate.
- ❖ STORAGE: Store covered containers in the refrigerator for up to 5 days

Nutrition: Total calories: 8 Total fat: 1g; Saturated fat: <1g; Sodium: 214mg; Carbohydrates: 17g; Fiber: 6g; Protein: 6g

54) CREAMY POLENTA AND CHIVES WITH PARMESAN

Cooking Time: 15 Minutes **Servings: 5**

Ingredients:

- 1 tsp olive oil
- ¼ cup minced shallot
- ½ cup white wine
- 3¼ cups water
- ¾ cup cornmeal
- 3 tbsp grated Parmesan cheese
- ½ tsp kosher salt
- ¼ cup chopped chives

Directions:

- Heat the oil in a saucepan over medium heat. Once the oil is shimmering, add the shallot and sauté for 2 minutes. Add the wine and water and bring to a boil.
- Pour the cornmeal in a thin, even stream into the liquid, stirring continuously until the mixture starts to thicken.
- Reduce the heat to low and continue to cook for 10 to 12 minutes, whisking every 1 to 2 minutes.
- Turn the heat off and stir in the cheese, salt, and chives. Cool.
- Place about ¾ cup of polenta in each of containers.
- STORAGE: Store covered containers in the refrigerator for up to 5 days.

Nutrition: Total calories: 110; Total fat: 3g; Saturated fat: 1g; Sodium: 29g; Carbohydrates: 16g; Fiber: 1g; Protein: 3g

55) SPECIAL MOCHA-NUT STUFFED DATES

Cooking Time: 10 Minutes **Servings: 5**

Ingredients:

- 2 tbsp creamy, unsweetened, unsalted almond butter
- 1 tsp unsweetened cocoa powder
- 3 tbsp walnut pieces
- 2 tbsp water
- ¼ tsp honey
- ¾ tsp instant espresso powder
- 10 Medjool dates, pitted

Directions:

- In a small bowl, combine the almond butter, cocoa powder, and walnut pieces.
- Place the water in a small microwaveable mug and heat on high for 30 seconds. Add the honey and espresso powder to the water and stir to dissolve.
- Add the espresso water to the cocoa bowl and combine thoroughly until a creamy, thick paste forms.
- Stuff each pitted date with 1 tsp of mocha filling.
- Place 2 dates in each of small containers.
- STORAGE: Store covered containers in the refrigerator for up to 5 days.

Nutrition: Total calories: 205; Total fat: ; Saturated fat: 1g; Sodium: 1mg; Carbohydrates: 39g; Fiber: 4g; Protein: 3g

56) EGGPLANT DIP ROAST (BABA GHANOUSH)

Cooking Time: 45 Minutes **Servings: 2 Cups**

Ingredients:

- 2 eggplants (close to 1 pound each)
- 1 tsp chopped garlic
- 3 tbsp unsalted tahini
- ¼ cup freshly squeezed lemon juice
- 1 tbsp olive oil
- ½ tsp kosher salt

Directions:

- Preheat the oven to 450°F and line a sheet pan with a silicone baking mat or parchment paper.
- Prick the eggplants in many places with a fork, place on the sheet pan, and roast in the oven until extremely soft, about 45 minutes. The eggplants should look like they are deflating.
- When the eggplants are cool, cut them open and scoop the flesh into a large bowl. You may need to use your hands to pull the flesh away from the skin. Discard the skin. Mash the flesh very well with a fork.
- Add the garlic, tahini, lemon juice, oil, and salt. Taste and adjust the seasoning with additional lemon juice, salt, or tahini if needed.
- Scoop the dip into a container and refrigerate.
- STORAGE: Store the covered container in the refrigerator for up to 5 days.

Nutrition: (¼ cup): Total calories: 8 Total fat: 5g; Saturated fat: 1g; Sodium: 156mg; Carbohydrates: 10g; Fiber: 4g; Protein: 2g

57) DELICIOUS HONEY-LEMON VINAIGRETTE

Cooking Time: 5 Minutes **Servings:** ½ Cup

Ingredients:

- ¼ cup freshly squeezed lemon juice
- 1 tsp honey
- 2 tsp Dijon mustard
- ⅛ tsp kosher salt
- ¼ cup olive oil

Directions:

- Place the lemon juice, honey, mustard, and salt in a small bowl and whisk to combine.
- Whisk in the oil, pouring it into the bowl in a thin steam.
- Pour the vinaigrette into a container and refrigerate.
- STORAGE: Store the covered container in the refrigerator for up to 2 weeks. Allow the vinaigrette to come to room temperature and shake before serving.

Nutrition: (2 tbsp): Total calories: 131; Total fat: 14g; Saturated fat: 2g; Sodium: 133mg; Carbohydrates: 3g; Fiber: <1g; Protein: <1g

58) SPANISH-STYLE ROMESCO SAUCE

Cooking Time: 10 Minutes **Servings:** 1⅔ Cups

Ingredients:

- ½ cup raw, unsalted almonds
- 4 medium garlic cloves (do not peel)
- 1 (12-ounce) jar of roasted red peppers, drained
- ½ cup canned diced fire-roasted tomatoes, drained
- 1 tsp smoked paprika
- ½ tsp kosher salt
- Pinch cayenne pepper
- 2 tsp red wine vinegar
- 2 tbsp olive oil

Directions:

- Preheat the oven to 350°F.
- Place the almonds and garlic cloves on a sheet pan and toast in the oven for 10 minutes. Remove from the oven and peel the garlic when cool enough to handle.
- Place the almonds in the bowl of a food processor. Process the almonds until they resemble coarse sand, to 45 seconds. Add the garlic, peppers, tomatoes, paprika, salt, and cayenne. Blend until smooth.
- Once the mixture is smooth, add the vinegar and oil and blend until well combined. Taste and add more vinegar or salt if needed.
- Scoop the romesco sauce into a container and refrigerate.
- STORAGE: Store the covered container in the refrigerator for up to 7 days.

Nutrition: (⅓ cup): Total calories: 158; Total fat: 13g; Saturated fat: 1g; Sodium: 292mg; Carbohydrates: 10g; Fiber: 3g; Protein: 4g

59) CARDAMOM MASCARPONE AND STRAWBERRIES

Cooking Time: 10 Minutes **Servings:** 4

Ingredients:

- 1 (8-ounce) container mascarpone cheese
- 2 tsp honey
- ¼ tsp ground cardamom
- 2 tbsp milk
- 1 pound strawberries (should be 24 strawberries in the pack)

Directions:

- Combine the mascarpone, honey, cardamom, and milk in a medium mixing bowl.
- Mix the ingredients with a spoon until super creamy, about 30 seconds.
- Place 6 strawberries and 2 tbsp of the mascarpone mixture in each of 4 containers.
- STORAGE: Store covered containers in the refrigerator for up to 5 days.

Nutrition: Total calories: 289; Total fat: 2; Saturated fat: 10g; Sodium: 26mg; Carbohydrates: 11g; Fiber: 3g; Protein: 1g

60) SWEET SPICY GREEN PUMPKIN SEEDS

Cooking Time: 15 Minutes **Servings:** 2 Cups

Ingredients:

- 2 cups raw green pumpkin seeds (pepitas)
- 1 egg white, beaten until frothy
- 3 tbsp honey
- 1 tbsp chili powder
- ¼ tsp cayenne pepper
- 1 tsp ground cinnamon
- ¼ tsp kosher salt

Directions:

- Preheat the oven to 350°F. Line a sheet pan with a silicone baking mat or parchment paper.
- In a medium bowl, mix all the ingredients until the seeds are well coated. Place on the lined sheet pan in a single, even layer.
- Bake for 15 minutes. Cool the seeds on the sheet pan, then peel clusters from the baking mat and break apart into small pieces.
- Place ¼ cup of seeds in each of 8 small containers or resealable sandwich bags.
- STORAGE: Store covered containers or resealable bags at room temperature for up to days.

Nutrition: (¼ cup): Total calories: 209; Total fat: 15g; Saturated fat: 3g; Sodium: 85mg; Carbohydrates: 11g; Fiber: 2g; Protein: 10g

61) DELICIOUS RASPBERRY RED WINE SAUCE

Cooking Time: 20 Minutes **Servings:** 1 Cup

Ingredients:

- ✓ 2 tsp olive oil
- ✓ 2 tbsp finely chopped shallot
- ✓ 1½ cups frozen raspberries
- ✓ 1 cup dry, fruity red wine

- ✓ 1 tsp thyme leaves, roughly chopped
- ✓ 1 tsp honey
- ✓ ¼ tsp kosher salt
- ✓ ½ tsp unsweetened cocoa powder

Directions:

- ❖ In a -inch skillet, heat the oil over medium heat. Add the shallot and cook until soft, about 2 minutes.
- ❖ Add the raspberries, wine, thyme, and honey and cook on medium heat until reduced, about 15 minutes. Stir in the salt and cocoa powder.
- ❖ Transfer the sauce to a blender and blend until smooth. Depending on how much you can scrape out of your blender, this recipe makes ¾ to 1 cup of sauce.
- ❖ Scoop the sauce into a container and refrigerate.
- ❖ STORAGE: Store the covered container in the refrigerator for up to 7 days.

Nutrition: (¼ cup): Total calories: 107; Total fat: 3g; Saturated fat: <1g; Sodium: 148mg; Carbohydrates: 1g; Fiber: 4g; Protein: 1g

62) ANTIPASTO SHRIMP SKEWERS

Cooking Time: 10 Minutes   **Servings: 4**

Ingredients:

- ✓ 16 pitted kalamata or green olives
- ✓ 16 fresh mozzarella balls (ciliegine)

- ✓ 16 cherry tomatoes
- ✓ 16 medium (41 to 50 per pound) precooked peeled, deveined shrimp
- ✓ 8 (8-inch) wooden or metal skewers

Directions:

- ❖ Alternate 2 olives, 2 mozzarella balls, 2 cherry tomatoes, and 2 shrimp on 8 skewers.
- ❖ Place skewers in each of 4 containers.
- ❖ STORAGE: Store covered containers in the refrigerator for up to 4 days.

Nutrition: Total calories: 108; Total fat: 6g; Saturated fat: 1g; Sodium: 328mg; Carbohydrates: ; Fiber: 1g; Protein: 9g

63) SMOKED PAPRIKA WITH OLIVE OIL–MARINATED CARROTS

Cooking Time: 5 Minutes   **Servings: 4**

Ingredients:

- ✓ 1 (1-pound) bag baby carrots (not the petite size)
- ✓ 2 tbsp olive oil
- ✓ 2 tbsp red wine vinegar
- ✓ ¼ tsp garlic powder
- ✓ ¼ tsp ground cumin

- ✓ ¼ tsp smoked paprika
- ✓ ⅛ tsp red pepper flakes
- ✓ ¼ cup chopped parsley
- ✓ ¼ tsp kosher salt

Directions:

- ❖ Pour enough water into a saucepan to come ¼ inch up the sides. Turn the heat to high, bring the water to a boil, add the carrots, and cover with a lid. Steam the carrots for 5 minutes, until crisp tender.
- ❖ After the carrots have cooled, mix with the oil, vinegar, garlic powder, cumin, paprika, red pepper, parsley, and salt.
- ❖ Place ¾ cup of carrots in each of 4 containers.
- ❖ STORAGE: Store covered containers in the refrigerator for up to 5 days.

Nutrition: Total calories: 109; Total fat: 7g; Saturated fat: 1g; Sodium: 234mg; Carbohydrates: 11g; Fiber: 3g; Protein: 2g

64) GREEK TZATZIKI SAUCE

Cooking Time: 15 Minutes   **Servings: 2½ Cups**

Ingredients:

- ✓ 1 English cucumber
- ✓ 2 cups low-fat (2%) plain Greek yogurt
- ✓ 1 tbsp olive oil
- ✓ 2 tsp freshly squeezed lemon juice
- ✓ ½ tsp chopped garlic

- ✓ ½ tsp kosher salt
- ✓ ⅛ tsp freshly ground black pepper
- ✓ 2 tbsp chopped fresh dill
- ✓ 2 tbsp chopped fresh mint

Directions:

- ❖ Place a sieve over a medium bowl. Grate the cucumber, with the skin, over the sieve. Press the grated cucumber into the sieve with the flat surface of a spatula to press as much liquid out as possible.
- ❖ In a separate medium bowl, place the yogurt, oil, lemon juice, garlic, salt, pepper, dill, and mint and stir to combine.
- ❖ Press on the cucumber one last time, then add it to the yogurt mixture. Stir to combine. Taste and add more salt and lemon juice if necessary.
- ❖ Scoop the sauce into a container and refrigerate.
- ❖ STORAGE: Store the covered container in the refrigerator for up to days.

Nutrition: (¼ cup): Total calories: 51; Total fat: 2g; Saturated fat: 1g; Sodium: 137mg; Carbohydrates: 3g; Fiber: <1g; Protein: 5g

Desserts & Snacks Recipes

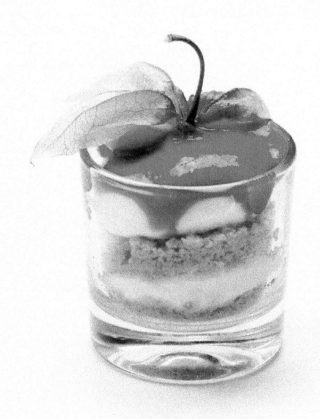

DESSERTS & SNACKS

65) CHERRY BROWNIES AND WALNUTS

Cooking Time: 25 To 30 Minutes   **Servings: 9**

Ingredients:

- ✓ 9 fresh cherries that are stemmed and pitted or 9 frozen cherries
- ✓ ½ cup sugar or sweetener substitute
- ✓ ¼ cup extra virgin olive oil
- ✓ 1 tsp vanilla extract
- ✓ ¼ tsp sea salt
- ✓ ½ cup whole-wheat pastry flour
- ✓ ¼ tsp baking powder
- ✓ ⅓ cup walnuts, chopped
- ✓ 2 eggs
- ✓ ½ cup plain Greek yogurt
- ✓ ⅓ cup cocoa powder, unsweetened

Directions:

- ❖ Make sure one of the metal racks in your oven is set in the middle.
- ❖ Turn the temperature on your oven to 375 degrees Fahrenheit.
- ❖ Using cooking spray, grease a 9-inch square pan.
- ❖ Take a large bowl and add the oil and sugar or sweetener substitute. Whisk the ingredients well.
- ❖ Add the eggs and use a mixer to beat the ingredients together.
- ❖ Pour in the yogurt and continue to beat the mixture until it is smooth.
- ❖ Take a medium bowl and combine the cocoa powder, flour, sea salt, and baking powder by whisking them together.
- ❖ Combine the powdered ingredients into the wet ingredients and use your electronic mixer to incorporate the ingredients together thoroughly.
- ❖ Add in the walnuts and stir.
- ❖ Pour the mixture into the pan.
- ❖ Sprinkle the cherries on top and push them into the batter. You can use any design, but it is best to make three rows and three columns with the cherries. This ensures that each piece of the brownie will have one cherry.
- ❖ Put the batter into the oven and turn your timer to 20 minutes.
- ❖ Check that the brownies are done using the toothpick test before removing them from the oven. Push the toothpick into the middle of the brownies and once it comes out clean, remove the brownies.
- ❖ Let the brownies cool for 5 to 10 minutes before cutting and serving.

Nutrition: calories: 225, fats: 10 grams, carbohydrates: 30 grams, protein: 5 grams

66) SPECIAL FRUIT DIP

Cooking Time: 10 To 15 Minutes   **Servings: 10**

Ingredients:

- ✓ ¼ cup coconut milk, full-fat is best
- ✓ ¼ cup vanilla yogurt
- ✓ ⅓ cup marshmallow creme
- ✓ 1 cup cream cheese, set at room temperature
- ✓ 2 tbsp maraschino cherry juice

Directions:

- ❖ In a large bowl, add the coconut milk, vanilla yogurt, marshmallow creme, cream cheese, and cherry juice.
- ❖ Using an electric mixer, set to low speed and blend the ingredients together until the fruit dip is smooth.
- ❖ Serve the dip with some of your favorite fruits and enjoy!

Nutrition: calories: 110, fats: 11 grams, carbohydrates: 3 grams, protein: 3 grams

67) DELICIOUS LEMONY TREAT

Cooking Time: 30 Minutes   **Servings: 4**

Ingredients:

- ✓ 1 lemon, medium in size
- ✓ 1 ½ tsp cornstarch
- ✓ 1 cup Greek yogurt, plain is best
- ✓ Fresh fruit
- ✓ ¼ cup cold water
- ✓ ⅔ cup heavy whipped cream
- ✓ 3 tbsp honey
- ✓ Optional: mint leaves

Directions:

- ❖ Take a large glass bowl and your metal, electric mixer and set them in the refrigerator so they can chill.
- ❖ In a separate bowl, add the yogurt and set that in the fridge.
- ❖ Zest the lemon into a medium bowl that is microwavable.
- ❖ Cut the lemon in half and then squeeze 1 tbsp of lemon juice into the bowl.
- ❖ Combine the cornstarch and water. Mix the ingredients thoroughly.
- ❖ Pour in the honey and whisk the ingredients together.
- ❖ Put the mixture into the microwave for 1 minute on high.
- ❖ Once the microwave stops, remove the mixture and stir.
- ❖ Set it back into the microwave for 15 to 30 seconds or until the mixture starts to bubble and thicken.
- ❖ Take the bowl of yogurt from the fridge and pour in the warm mixture while whisking.
- ❖ Put the yogurt mixture back into the fridge.
- ❖ Take the large bowl and beaters out of the fridge.
- ❖ Put your electronic mixer together and pour the whipped cream into the chilled bowl.
- ❖ Beat the cream until soft peaks start to form. This can take up to 3 minutes, depending on how fresh your cream is.
- ❖ Remove the yogurt from the fridge.
- ❖ Fold the yogurt into the cream using a rubber spatula. Remember to lift and turn the mixture so it doesn't deflate.
- ❖ Place back into the fridge until you are serving the dessert or for 15 minutes. The dessert should not be in the fridge for longer than 1 hour.
- ❖ When you serve the lemony goodness, you will spoon it into four dessert dishes and drizzle with extra honey or even melt some chocolate to drizzle on top.
- ❖ Add a little fresh mint and enjoy!

Nutrition: calories: 241, fats: 16 grams, carbohydrates: 21 grams, protein: 7 grams

68) MELON AND GINGER

Cooking Time: 10 To 15 Minutes   **Servings: 4**

Ingredients:

- ✓ ½ cantaloupe, cut into 1-inch chunks
- ✓ 2 cups of watermelon, cut into 1-inch chunks
- ✓ 2 cups honeydew melon, cut into 1-inch chunks
- ✓ 2 tbsp of raw honey
- ✓ Ginger, 2 inches in size, peeled, grated, and preserve the juice

Directions:

- ❖ In a large bowl, combine your cantaloupe, honeydew melon, and watermelon. Gently mix the ingredients.
- ❖ Combine the ginger juice and stir.
- ❖ Drizzle on the honey, serve, and enjoy! You can also chill the mixture for up to an hour before serving.

Nutrition: calories: 91, fats: 0 grams, carbohydrates: 23 grams, protein: 1 gram.

69) DELICIOUS ALMOND SHORTBREAD COOKIES

Cooking Time: 25 Minutes   **Servings: 16**

Ingredients:

- ½ cup coconut oil
- 1 tsp vanilla extract
- 2 egg yolks
- 1 tbsp brandy
- 1 cup powdered sugar
- 1 cup finely ground almonds
- 3 ½ cups cake flour
- ½ cup almond butter
- 1 tbsp water or rose flower water

Directions:

- In a large bowl, combine the coconut oil, powdered sugar, and butter. If the butter is not soft, you want to wait until it softens up. Use an electric mixer to beat the ingredients together at high speed.
- In a small bowl, add the egg yolks, brandy, water, and vanilla extract. Whisk well.
- Fold the egg yolk mixture into the large bowl.
- Add the flour and almonds. Fold and mix with a wooden spoon.
- Place the mixture into the fridge for at least 1 hour and 30 minutes.
- Preheat your oven to 325 degrees Fahrenheit.
- Take the mixture, which now looks like dough, and divide it into 1-inch balls.
- With a piece of parchment paper on a baking sheet, arrange the cookies and flatten them with a fork or your fingers.
- Place the cookies in the oven for 13 minutes, but watch them so they don't burn.
- Transfer the cookies onto a rack to cool for a couple of minutes before enjoying!

Nutrition: calories: 250, fats: 14 grams, carbohydrates: 30 grams, protein: 3 grams

70) CLASSIC CHOCOLATE FRUIT KEBABS

Cooking Time: 30 Minutes   **Servings: 6**

Ingredients:

- 24 blueberries
- 12 strawberries with the green leafy top part removed
- 12 green or red grapes, seedless
- 12 pitted cherries
- 8 ounces chocolate

Directions:

- Line a baking sheet with a piece of parchment paper and place 6, -inch long wooden skewers on top of the paper.
- Start by threading a piece of fruit onto the skewers. You can create and follow any pattern that you like with the ingredients. An example pattern is 1 strawberry, 1 cherry, blueberries, 2 grapes. Repeat the pattern until all of the fruit is on the skewers.
- In a saucepan on medium heat, melt the chocolate. Stir continuously until the chocolate has melted completely.
- Carefully scoop the chocolate into a plastic sandwich bag and twist the bag closed starting right above the chocolate.
- Snip the corner of the bag with scissors.
- Drizzle the chocolate onto the kebabs by squeezing it out of the bag.
- Put the baking pan into the freezer for 20 minutes.
- Serve and enjoy!

Nutrition: calories: 254, fats: 15 grams, carbohydrates: 28 grams, protein: 4 grams.*71)*

72) PEACHES AND BLUE CHEESE CREAM

Cooking Time: 20 Hours 10 Minutes   **Servings: 4**

Ingredients:

- 4 peaches
- 1 cinnamon stick
- 4 ounces sliced blue cheese
- ⅓ cup orange juice, freshly squeezed is best
- 3 whole cloves
- 1 tsp of orange zest, taken from the orange peel
- ¼ tsp cardamom pods
- ⅔ cup red wine
- 2 tbsp honey, raw or your preferred variety
- 1 vanilla bean
- 1 tsp allspice berries
- 4 tbsp dried cherries

Directions:

- Set a saucepan on top of your stove range and add the cinnamon stick, cloves, orange juice, cardamom, vanilla, allspice, red wine, and orange zest. Whisk the ingredients well. Add your peaches to the mixture and poach them for hours or until they become soft.
- Take a spoon to remove the peaches and boil the rest of the liquid to make the syrup. You want the liquid to reduce itself by at least half.
- While the liquid is boiling, combine the dried cherries, blue cheese, and honey into a bowl. Once your peaches are cooled, slice them into halves.
- Top each peach with the blue cheese mixture and then drizzle the liquid onto the top. Serve and enjoy!

Nutrition: calories: 211, fats: 24 grams, carbohydrates: 15 grams, protein: 6 grams

73) MEDITERRANEAN-STYLE BLACKBERRY ICE CREAM

Cooking Time: 15 Minutes   **Servings:** 6

Ingredients:

- 3 egg yolks
- 1 container of Greek yogurt
- 1 pound mashed blackberries
- ½ tsp vanilla essence
- 1 tsp arrowroot powder
- ¼ tsp ground cloves
- 5 ounces sugar or sweetener substitute
- 1 pound heavy cream

Directions:

- In a small bowl, add the arrowroot powder and egg yolks. Whisk or beat them with an electronic mixture until they are well combined.
- Set a saucepan on top of your stove and turn your heat to medium.
- Add the heavy cream and bring it to a boil.
- Turn off the heat and add the egg mixture into the cream through folding.
- Turn the heat back on to medium and pour in the sugar. Cook the mixture for 10 minutes or until it starts to thicken.
- Remove the mixture from heat and place it in the fridge so it can completely cool. This should take about one hour.
- Once the mixture is cooled, add in the Greek yogurt, ground cloves, blackberries, and vanilla by folding in the ingredients.
- Transfer the ice cream into a container and place it in the freezer for at least two hours.
- Serve and enjoy!

Nutrition: calories: 402, fats: 20 grams, carbohydrates: 52 grams, protein: 8 grams

74) CLASSIC STUFFED FIGS

Cooking Time: 20 Minutes   **Servings:** 6

Ingredients:

- 10 halved fresh figs
- 20 chopped almonds
- 4 ounces goat cheese, divided
- 2 tbsp of raw honey

Directions:

- Turn your oven to broiler mode and set it to a high temperature.
- Place your figs, cut side up, on a baking sheet. If you like to place a piece of parchment paper on top you can do this, but it is not necessary.
- Sprinkle each fig with half of the goat cheese.
- Add a tbsp of chopped almonds to each fig.
- Broil the figs for 3 to 4 minutes.
- Take them out of the oven and let them cool for 5 to 7 minutes.
- Sprinkle with the remaining goat cheese and honey.

Nutrition: calories: 209, fats: 9 grams, carbohydrates: 26 grams, protein: grams.

75) CHIA PUDDING AND STRAWBERRIES

Cooking Time: 4 Hours 5 Minutes   **Servings:** 4

Ingredients:

- 2 cups unsweetened almond milk
- 1 tbsp vanilla extract
- 2 tbsp raw honey
- ¼ cup chia seeds
- 2 cups fresh and sliced strawberries

Directions:

- In a medium bowl, combine the honey, chia seeds, vanilla, and unsweetened almond milk. Mix well.
- Set the mixture in the refrigerator for at least 4 hours.
- When you serve the pudding, top it with strawberries. You can even create a design in a glass serving bowl or dessert dish by adding a little pudding on the bottom, a few strawberries, top the strawberries with some more pudding, and then top the dish with a few strawberries.

Nutrition: calories: 108, fats: grams, carbohydrates: 17 grams, protein: 3 grams

Meat Recipes

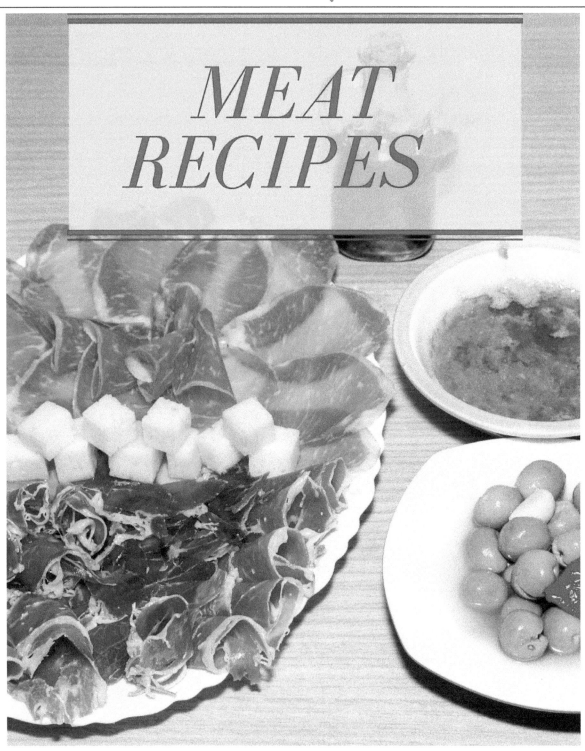

76) CLASSIC AIOLI BAKED CHICKEN WINGS

Cooking Time: 35 Minutes   **Servings:** 4

Ingredients:

- ✓ 4 chicken wings
- ✓ 1 cup Halloumi cheese, cubed
- ✓ 1 tbsp garlic, finely minced
- ✓ 1 tbsp fresh lime juice
- ✓ 1 tbsp fresh coriander, chopped
- ✓ 6 black olives, pitted and halved
- ✓ 1 ½ tbsp butter
- ✓ 1 hard-boiled egg yolk
- ✓ 1 tbsp balsamic vinegar
- ✓ 1/2 cup extra-virgin olive oil
- ✓ 1/4 tsp flaky sea salt
- ✓ Sea salt and pepper, to season

Directions:

- ❖ In a saucepan, melt the butter until sizzling. Sear the chicken wings for 5 minutes per side. Season with salt and pepper to taste.
- ❖ Place the chicken wings on a parchment-lined baking pan
- ❖ Mix the egg yolk, garlic, lime juice, balsamic vinegar, olive oil, and salt in your blender until creamy, uniform and smooth.
- ❖ Spread the Aioli over the fried chicken. Now, scatter the coriander and black olives on top of the chicken wings.
- ❖ Bake in the preheated oven at 380 degrees F for 20 to 2minutes. Top with the cheese and bake an additional 5 minutes until hot and bubbly.
- ❖ Storing
- ❖ Place the chicken wings in airtight containers or Ziploc bags; keep in your refrigerator for up 3 to 4 days.
- ❖ For freezing, place the chicken wings in airtight containers or heavy-duty freezer bags. Freeze up to 3 months. Once thawed in the refrigerator, heat in the preheated oven at 375 degrees F for 20 to 25 minutes or until heated through. Enjoy!

Nutrition: 562 Calories; 43.8g Fat; 2.1g Carbs; 40.8g Protein; 0.4g Fiber

77) SPECIAL SMOKED PORK SAUSAGE KETO BOMBS

Cooking Time: 15 Minutes   **Servings:** 6

Ingredients:

- ✓ 3/4 pound smoked pork sausage, ground
- ✓ 1 tsp ginger-garlic paste
- ✓ 2 tbsp scallions, minced
- ✓ 1 tbsp butter, room temperature
- ✓ 1 tomato, pureed
- ✓ 4 ounces mozzarella cheese, crumbled
- ✓ 2 tbsp flaxseed meal
- ✓ 8 ounces cream cheese, room temperature
- ✓ Sea salt and ground black pepper, to taste

Directions:

- ❖ Melt the butter in a frying pan over medium-high heat. Cook the sausage for about 4 minutes, crumbling with a spatula.
- ❖ Add in the ginger-garlic paste, scallions, and tomato; continue to cook over medium-low heat for a further 6 minutes. Stir in the remaining ingredients.
- ❖ Place the mixture in your refrigerator for 1 to 2 hours until firm. Roll the mixture into bite-sized balls.
- ❖ Storing
- ❖ Transfer the balls to the airtight containers and place in your refrigerator for up to 3 days.
- ❖ For freezing, place in a freezer safe containers and freeze up to 1 month. Enjoy!

Nutrition: 383 Calories; 32. Fat; 5.1g Carbs; 16.7g Protein; 1.7g Fiber

78) TURKEY MEATBALLS AND TANGY BASIL CHUTNEY

Cooking Time: 30 Minutes   **Servings:** 6

Ingredients:

- ✓ 2 tbsp sesame oil
- ✓ For the Meatballs:
- ✓ 1/2 cup Romano cheese, grated
- ✓ 1 tsp garlic, minced
- ✓ 1/2 tsp shallot powder
- ✓ 1/4 tsp dried thyme
- ✓ 1/2 tsp mustard seeds
- ✓ 2 small-sized eggs, lightly beaten
- ✓ 1 ½ pounds ground turkey
- ✓ 1/2 tsp sea salt
- ✓ 1/4 tsp ground black pepper, or more to taste
- ✓ 3 tbsp almond meal
- ✓ For the Basil Chutney:
- ✓ 2 tbsp fresh lime juice
- ✓ 1/4 cup fresh basil leaves
- ✓ 1/4 cup fresh parsley
- ✓ 1/2 cup cilantro leaves
- ✓ 1 tsp fresh ginger root, grated
- ✓ 2 tbsp olive oil
- ✓ 2 tbsp water
- ✓ 1 tbsp habanero chili pepper, deveined and minced

Directions:

- ❖ In a mixing bowl, combine all ingredients for the meatballs. Roll the mixture into meatballs and reserve.
- ❖ Heat the sesame oil in a frying pan over a moderate flame. Sear the meatballs for about 8 minutes until browned on all sides.
- ❖ Make the chutney by mixing all the ingredients in your blender or food processor.
- ❖ Storing
- ❖ Place the meatballs in airtight containers or Ziploc bags; keep in your refrigerator for up to 3 to 4 days.
- ❖ Freeze the meatballs in airtight containers or heavy-duty freezer bags. Freeze up to 3 to 4 months. To defrost, slowly reheat in a frying pan.
- ❖ Store the basil chutney in the refrigerator for up to a week. Bon appétit!

Nutrition: 390 Calories; 27.2g Fat; 1. Carbs; 37.4g Protein; 0.3g Fiber

79) ROASTED CHICKEN AND CASHEW PESTO

Cooking Time: 35 Minutes   **Servings:** 4

Ingredients:

- ✓ 1 cup leeks, chopped
- ✓ 1 pound chicken legs, skinless
- ✓ Salt and ground black pepper, to taste
- ✓ 1/2 tsp red pepper flakes
- ✓ For the Cashew-Basil Pesto:

- ✓ 1/2 cup cashews
- ✓ 2 garlic cloves, minced
- ✓ 1/2 cup fresh basil leaves
- ✓ 1/2 cup Parmigiano-Reggiano cheese, preferably freshly grated
- ✓ 1/2 cup olive oil

Directions:

- ❖ Place the chicken legs in a parchment-lined baking pan. Season with salt and pepper, Then, scatter the leeks around the chicken legs.
- ❖ Roast in the preheated oven at 390 degrees F for 30 to 35 minutes, rotating the pan occasionally.
- ❖ Pulse the cashews, basil, garlic, and cheese in your blender until pieces are small. Continue blending while adding olive oil to the mixture. Mix until the desired consistency is reached.
- ❖ Storing
- ❖ Place the chicken in airtight containers or Ziploc bags; keep in your refrigerator for up 3 to 4 days.
- ❖ To freeze the chicken legs, place them in airtight containers or heavy-duty freezer bags. Freeze up to 3 months. Once thawed in the refrigerator, heat in the preheated oven at 375 degrees F for 20 to 25 minutes.
- ❖ Store your pesto in the refrigerator for up to a week. Bon appétit!

Nutrition: 5 Calories; 44.8g Fat; 5g Carbs; 38.7g Protein; 1g Fiber

80) SPECIAL DUCK BREASTS IN BOOZY SAUCE

Cooking Time: 20 Minutes   **Servings:** 4

Ingredients:

- ✓ 1 ½ pounds duck breasts, butterflied
- ✓ 1 tbsp tallow, room temperature
- ✓ 1 ½ cups chicken consommé
- ✓ 3 tbsp soy sauce

- ✓ 2 ounces vodka
- ✓ 1/2 cup sour cream
- ✓ 4 scallion stalks, chopped
- ✓ Salt and pepper, to taste

Directions:

- ❖ Melt the tallow in a frying pan over medium-high flame. Sear the duck breasts for about 5 minutes, flipping them over occasionally to ensure even cooking.
- ❖ Add in the scallions, salt, pepper, chicken consommé, and soy sauce. Partially cover and continue to cook for a further 8 minutes.
- ❖ Add in the vodka and sour cream; remove from the heat and stir to combine well.
- ❖ Storing
- ❖ Place the duck breasts in airtight containers or Ziploc bags; keep in your refrigerator for up to 3 to 4 days.
- ❖ For freezing, place duck breasts in airtight containers or heavy-duty freezer bags. Freeze up to 2 to 3 months. Once thawed in the refrigerator, reheat in a saucepan. Bon appétit!

Nutrition: 351 Calories; 24. Fat; 6.6g Carbs; 22.1g Protein; 0.6g Fiber

81) WHITE CAULIFLOWER WITH CHICKEN CHOWDER

Cooking Time: 30 Minutes   **Servings:** 6

Ingredients:

- ✓ 1 cup leftover roast chicken breasts
- ✓ 1 head cauliflower, broken into small-sized florets
- ✓ Sea salt and ground white pepper, to taste
- ✓ 2 ½ cups water
- ✓ 3 cups chicken consommé

- ✓ 1 ¼ cups sour cream
- ✓ 1/2 stick butter
- ✓ 1/2 cup white onion, finely chopped
- ✓ 1 tsp fresh garlic, finely minced
- ✓ 1 celery, chopped

Directions:

- ❖ In a heavy bottomed pot, melt the butter over a moderate heat. Cook the onion, garlic and celery for about 5 minutes or until they've softened.
- ❖ Add in the salt, white pepper, water, chicken consommé, chicken, and cauliflower florets; bring to a boil. Reduce the temperature to simmer and continue to cook for 30 minutes.
- ❖ Puree the soup with an immersion blender. Fold in sour cream and stir to combine well.
- ❖ Storing
- ❖ Spoon your chowder into airtight containers or Ziploc bags; keep in your refrigerator for up to 3 to 4 days.
- ❖ For freezing, place your chowder in airtight containers. It will maintain the best quality for about 4 to months. Defrost in the refrigerator. Bon appétit!

Nutrition: 231 Calories; 18.2g Fat; 5.9g Carbs; 11.9g Protein; 1.4g Fiber

82) Taro Leaf with Chicken Soup

Cooking Time: 45 Minutes   **Servings:** 4

Ingredients:

- ✓ 1 pound whole chicken, boneless and chopped into small chunks
- ✓ 1/2 cup onions, chopped
- ✓ 1/2 cup rutabaga, cubed
- ✓ 2 carrots, peeled
- ✓ 2 celery stalks
- ✓ Salt and black pepper, to taste
- ✓ 1 cup chicken bone broth
- ✓ 1/2 tsp ginger-garlic paste
- ✓ 1/2 cup taro leaves, roughly chopped
- ✓ 1 tbsp fresh coriander, chopped
- ✓ 3 cups water
- ✓ 1 tsp paprika

Directions:

- ❖ Place all ingredients in a heavy-bottomed pot. Bring to a boil over the highest heat.
- ❖ Turn the heat to simmer. Continue to cook, partially covered, an additional 40 minutes.
- ❖ Storing
- ❖ Spoon the soup into four airtight containers or Ziploc bags; keep in your refrigerator for up to 3 to days.
- ❖ For freezing, place the soup in airtight containers. It will maintain the best quality for about to 6 months. Defrost in the refrigerator. Bon appétit!

Nutrition: 25Calories; 12.9g Fat; 3.2g Carbs; 35.1g Protein; 2.2g Fiber

83) CREAMY GREEK-STYLE SOUP

Cooking Time: 30 Minutes **Servings: 4**

Ingredients:

- ✓ 1/2 stick butter
- ✓ 1/2 cup zucchini, diced
- ✓ 2 garlic cloves, minced
- ✓ 4 ½ cups roasted vegetable broth
- ✓ Sea salt and ground black pepper, to season
- ✓ 1 ½ cups leftover turkey, shredded
- ✓ 1/3 cup double cream
- ✓ 1/2 cup Greek-style yogurt

Directions:

- ❖ In a heavy-bottomed pot, melt the butter over medium-high heat. Once hot, cook the zucchini and garlic for 2 minutes until they are fragrant.
- ❖ Add in the broth, salt, black pepper, and leftover turkey. Cover and cook for minutes, stirring periodically.
- ❖ Then, fold in the cream and yogurt. Continue to cook for 5 minutes more or until thoroughly warmed.
- ❖ Storing
- ❖ Spoon the soup into four airtight containers or Ziploc bags; keep in your refrigerator for up to 3 to 4 days.
- ❖ For freezing, place the soup in airtight containers. It will maintain the best quality for about 4 to months. Defrost in the refrigerator. Enjoy!

Nutrition: 256 Calories; 18.8g Fat; 5.4g Carbs; 15.8g Protein; 0.2g Fiber

84) LOW-CARB PORK WRAPS

Cooking Time: 15 Minutes **Servings: 4**

Ingredients:

- ✓ 1 pound ground pork
- ✓ 2 garlic cloves, finely minced
- ✓ 1 chili pepper, deveined and finely minced
- ✓ 1 tsp mustard powder
- ✓ 1 tbsp sunflower seeds
- ✓ 2 tbsp champagne vinegar
- ✓ 1 tbsp coconut aminos
- ✓ Celery salt and ground black pepper, to taste
- ✓ 2 scallion stalks, sliced
- ✓ 1 head lettuce

Directions:

- ❖ Sear the ground pork in the preheated pan for about 8 minutes. Stir in the garlic, chili pepper, mustard seeds, and sunflower seeds; continue to sauté for minute longer or until aromatic.
- ❖ Add in the vinegar, coconut aminos, salt, black pepper, and scallions. Stir to combine well.
- ❖ Storing
- ❖ Place the ground pork mixture in airtight containers or Ziploc bags; keep in your refrigerator for up to 3 to days.
- ❖ For freezing, place the ground pork mixture it in airtight containers or heavy-duty freezer bags. Freeze up to 2 to 3 months. Defrost in the refrigerator and reheat in the skillet.
- ❖ Add spoonfuls of the pork mixture to the lettuce leaves, wrap them and serve.

Nutrition: 281 Calories; 19.4g Fat; 5.1g Carbs; 22.1g Protein; 1.3g Fiber

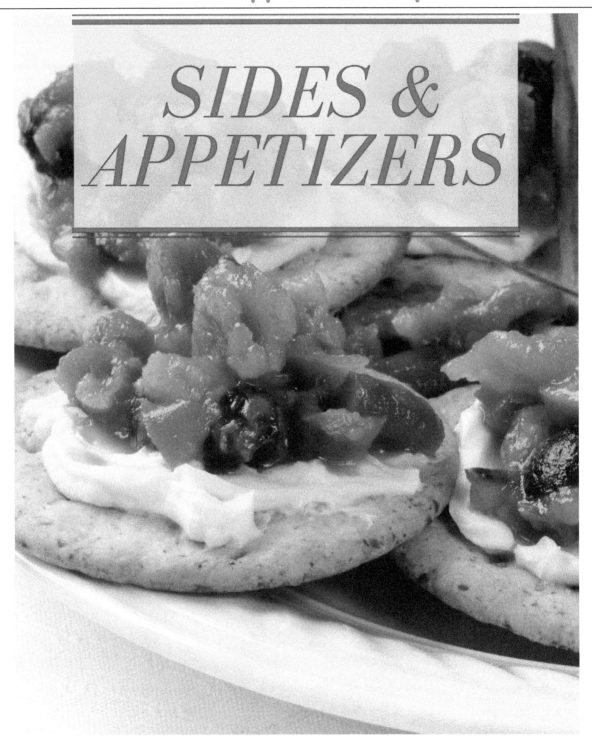

SIDES &
APPETIZERS

85) ITALIAN CHICKEN BACON PASTA

Cooking Time: 35 Minutes   **Servings: 4**

Ingredients:

- ✓ 8 ounces linguine pasta
- ✓ 3 slices of bacon
- ✓ 1 pound boneless chicken breast, cooked and diced
- ✓ Salt
- ✓ 1 6-ounce can artichoke hearts

- ✓ 2 ounce can diced tomatoes, undrained
- ✓ ¼ tsp dried rosemary
- ✓ 1/3 cup crumbled feta cheese, plus extra for topping
- ✓ 2/3 cup pitted black olives

Directions:

- ❖ Fill a large pot with salted water and bring to a boil.
- ❖ Add linguine and cook for 8-10 minutes until al dente.
- ❖ Cook bacon until brown, and then crumble.
- ❖ Season chicken with salt.
- ❖ Place chicken and bacon into a large skillet.
- ❖ Add tomatoes and rosemary and simmer the mixture for about 20 minutes.
- ❖ Stir in feta cheese, artichoke hearts, and olives, and cook until thoroughly heated.
- ❖ Toss the freshly cooked pasta with chicken mixture and cool.
- ❖ Spread over the containers.
- ❖ Before eating, garnish with extra feta if your heart desires!

Nutrition: 755, Total Fat: 22.5 g, Saturated Fat: 6.5 g, Cholesterol: 128 mg, Sodium: 852 mg, Total Carbohydrate: 75.4 g, Dietary Fiber: 7.3 g, Total Sugars: 3.4 g, Protein: 55.6 g, Vitamin D: 0 mcg, Calcium: 162 mg, Iron: 7 mg, Potassium: 524 mg

86) LOVELY CREAMY GARLIC SHRIMP PASTA

Cooking Time: 15 Minutes   **Servings: 4**

Ingredients:

- ✓ 6 ounces whole-wheat spaghetti, your favorite
- ✓ 12 ounces raw shrimp, peeled, deveined, and cut into 1-inch pieces
- ✓ 1 bunch asparagus, trimmed and thinly sliced
- ✓ 1 large bell pepper, thinly sliced
- ✓ 3 cloves garlic, chopped

- ✓ 1¼ tsp kosher salt
- ✓ 1½ cups non-fat plain yogurt
- ✓ ¼ cup flat-leaf parsley, chopped
- ✓ 3 tbsp lemon juice
- ✓ 1 tbsp extra virgin olive oil
- ✓ ½ tsp fresh ground black pepper
- ✓ ¼ cup toasted pine nuts

Directions:

- ❖ Bring water to a boil in a large pot.
- ❖ Add spaghetti and cook for about minutes less than called for by the package instructions.
- ❖ Add shrimp, bell pepper, asparagus and cook for about 2-4 minutes until the shrimp are tender.
- ❖ Drain the pasta.
- ❖ In a large bowl, mash the garlic until paste forms.
- ❖ Whisk yogurt, parsley, oil, pepper, and lemon juice into the garlic paste.
- ❖ Add pasta mixture and toss well.
- ❖ Cool and spread over the containers.
- ❖ Sprinkle with pine nuts.
- ❖ Enjoy!

Nutrition: 504, Total Fat: 15.4 g, Saturated Fat: 4.9 g, Cholesterol: 199 mg, Sodium: 2052 mg, Total Carbohydrate: 42.2 g, Dietary Fiber: 3.5 g, Total Sugars: 26.6 g, Protein: 43.2 g, Vitamin D: 0 mcg, Calcium: 723 mg, Iron: 3 mg, Potassium: 3 mg

87) SPECIAL MUSHROOM FETTUCCINE

Cooking Time: 15 Minutes   **Servings: 5**

Ingredients:

- ✓ 12 ounces whole-wheat fettuccine (or any other)
- ✓ 1 tbsp extra virgin olive oil
- ✓ 4 cups mixed mushrooms, such as oyster, cremini, etc., sliced
- ✓ 4 cups broccoli, divided
- ✓ 1 tbsp minced garlic

- ✓ ½ cup dry sherry
- ✓ 2 cups low-fat milk
- ✓ 2 tbsp all-purpose flour
- ✓ ½ tsp salt
- ✓ ½ tsp freshly ground pepper
- ✓ 1 cup finely shredded Asiago cheese, plus some for topping

Directions:

- ❖ Cook pasta in a large pot of boiling water for about 8- minutes.
- ❖ Drain pasta and set it to the side. Add oil to large skillet and heat over medium heat.
- ❖ Add mushrooms and broccoli, and cook for about 8-10 minutes until the mushrooms have released the liquid.
- ❖ Add garlic and cook for about 1 minute until fragrant. Add sherry, making sure to scrape up any brown bits.
- ❖ Bring the mix to a boil and cook for about 1 minute until evaporated.
- ❖ In a separate bowl, whisk flour and milk. Add the mix to your skillet, and season with salt and pepper.
- ❖ Cook well for about 2 minutes until the sauce begins to bubble and is thickened. Stir in Asiago cheese until it has fully melted.
- ❖ Add the sauce to your pasta and give it a gentle toss. Spread over the containers. Serve with extra cheese.

Nutrition: 503, Total Fat: 19.6 g, Saturated Fat: 6.3 g, Cholesterol: 25 mg, Sodium: 1136 mg, Total Carbohydrate: 57.5 g, Dietary Fiber: 12.4 g, Total Sugars: 6.4 g, Protein: 24.5 g, Vitamin D: 51 mcg, Calcium: 419 mg, Iron: 5 mg, Potassium: 390 mg

88) ORIGINAL LEMON GARLIC SARDINE FETTUCCINE

Cooking Time: 15 Minutes   **Servings: 4**

Ingredients:

- ✓ 8 ounces whole-wheat fettuccine
- ✓ 4 tbsp extra-virgin olive oil, divided
- ✓ 4 cloves garlic, minced
- ✓ 1 cup fresh breadcrumbs
- ✓ ¼ cup lemon juice
- ✓ 1 tsp freshly ground pepper
- ✓ ½ tsp of salt
- ✓ 2 4-ounce cans boneless and skinless sardines, dipped in tomato sauce
- ✓ ½ cup fresh parsley, chopped
- ✓ ¼ cup finely shredded parmesan cheese

Directions:

- ❖ Fill a large pot with water and bring to a boil.
- ❖ Cook pasta according to package instructions until tender (about 10 minutes).
- ❖ In a small skillet, heat 2 tbsp of oil over medium heat.
- ❖ Add garlic and cook for about 20 seconds, until sizzling and fragrant.
- ❖ Transfer the garlic to a large bowl.
- ❖ Add the remaining 2 tbsp of oil to skillet and heat over medium heat.
- ❖ Add breadcrumbs and cook for 5-6 minutes until golden and crispy.
- ❖ Whisk lemon juice, salt, and pepper into the garlic bowl.
- ❖ Add pasta to the garlic bowl, along with garlic, sardines, parmesan, and parsley; give it a gentle stir.
- ❖ Cool and spread over the containers.
- ❖ Before eating, sprinkle with breadcrumbs.
- ❖ Enjoy!

Nutrition: 633, Total Fat: 27.7 g, Saturated Fat: 6.4 g, Cholesterol: 40 mg, Sodium: 771 mg, Total Carbohydrate: 55.9 g, Dietary Fiber: 7.7 g, Total Sugars: 2.1 g, Protein: 38.6 g, Vitamin D: 0 mcg, Calcium: 274 mg, Iron: 7 mg, Potassium: mg

89) DELICIOUS SPINACH ALMOND STIR-FRY

Cooking Time: 10 Minutes   **Servings: 2**

Ingredients:

- ✓ 2 ounces spinach
- ✓ 1 tbsp coconut oil
- ✓ 3 tbsp almond, slices
- ✓ sea salt or plain salt
- ✓ freshly ground black pepper

Directions:

- ❖ Start by heating a skillet with coconut oil; add spinach and let it cook.
- ❖ Then, add salt and pepper as the spinach is cooking.
- ❖ Finally, add in the almond slices.
- ❖ Serve warm.

Nutrition: 117, Total Fat: 11.4 g, Saturated Fat: 6.2 g, Cholesterol: 0 mg, Sodium: 23 mg, Total Carbohydrate: 2.9 g, Dietary Fiber: 1.7 g, Total Sugars: 0.g, Protein: 2.7 g, Vitamin D: 0 mcg, Calcium: 52 mg, Iron: 1 mg, Potassium: 224 mg

90) ITALIAN BBQ CARROTS

Cooking Time: 30 Minutes   **Servings: 8**

Ingredients:

- ✓ 2 pounds baby carrots (organic)
- ✓ 1 tbsp olive oil
- ✓ 1 tbsp garlic powder
- ✓ 1 tbsp onion powder
- ✓ sea salt or plain salt
- ✓ freshly ground black pepper

Directions:

- ❖ Mix all the Ingredients: in a plastic bag so that the carrots are well coated with the mixture.
- ❖ Then, on the BBQ grill place a piece of aluminum foil and spread the carrots in a single layer.
- ❖ Finally, grill for 30 minutes or until tender.
- ❖ Serve warm.

Nutrition: 388, Total Fat: 1.9 g, Saturated Fat: 0.3 g, Cholesterol: 0 mg, Sodium: 89 mg, Total Carbohydrate: 10.8 g, Dietary Fiber: 3.4 g, Total Sugars: 6 g, Protein: 1 g, Vitamin D: 0 mcg, Calcium: 40 mg, Iron: 1 mg, Potassium: 288 mg

91) MEDITERRANEAN-STYLE BAKED ZUCCHINI STICKS

Cooking Time: 20 Minutes **Servings:** 8

Ingredients:

- ✓ ¼ cup feta cheese, crumbled
- ✓ 4 zucchini
- ✓ ¼ cup parsley, chopped
- ✓ ½ cup tomatoes, minced
- ✓ ½ cup kalamata olives, pitted and minced
- ✓ 1 cup red bell pepper, minced
- ✓ 1 tbsp oregano
- ✓ ¼ cup garlic, minced
- ✓ 1 tbsp basil
- ✓ sea salt or plain salt
- ✓ freshly ground black pepper

Directions:

- ❖ Start by cutting zucchini in half (lengthwise) and scoop out the middle.
- ❖ Then, combine garlic, black pepper, bell pepper, oregano, basil, tomatoes, and olives in a bowl.
- ❖ Now, fill in the middle of each zucchini with this mixture. Place these on a prepared baking dish and bake the dish at 0 degrees F for about 15 minutes.
- ❖ Finally, top with feta cheese and broil on high for 3 minutes or until done. Garnish with parsley.
- ❖ Serve warm.

Nutrition: 53, Total Fat: 2.2 g, Saturated Fat: 0.9 g, Cholesterol: 4 mg, Sodium: 138 mg, Total Carbohydrate: 7.5 g, Dietary Fiber: 2.1 g, Total Sugars: 3 g, Protein: 2.g, Vitamin D: 0 mcg, Calcium: 67 mg, Iron: 1 mg, Potassium: 353 mg

92) ARTICHOKE OLIVE PASTA

Cooking Time: 25 Minutes **Servings:** 4

Ingredients:

- ✓ salt
- ✓ pepper
- ✓ 2 tbsp olive oil, divided
- ✓ 2 garlic cloves, thinly sliced
- ✓ 1 can artichoke hearts, drained, rinsed, and quartered lengthwise
- ✓ 1-pint grape tomatoes, halved lengthwise, divided
- ✓ ½ cup fresh basil leaves, torn apart
- ✓ 12 ounces whole-wheat spaghetti
- ✓ ½ medium onion, thinly sliced
- ✓ ½ cup dry white wine
- ✓ 1/3 cup pitted Kalamata olives, quartered lengthwise
- ✓ ¼ cup grated Parmesan cheese, plus extra for serving

Directions:

- ❖ Fill a large pot with salted water.
- ❖ Pour the water to a boil and cook your pasta according to package instructions until al dente.
- ❖ Drain the pasta and reserve 1 cup of the cooking water.
- ❖ Return the pasta to the pot and set aside.
- ❖ Heat 1 tbsp of olive oil in a large skillet over medium-high heat.
- ❖ Add onion and garlic, season with pepper and salt, and cook well for about 3-4 minutes until nicely browned.
- ❖ Add wine and cook for 2 minutes until evaporated.
- ❖ Stir in artichokes and keep cooking 2-3 minutes until brown.
- ❖ Add olives and half of your tomatoes.
- ❖ Cook well for 1-2 minutes until the tomatoes start to break down.
- ❖ Add pasta to the skillet.
- ❖ Stir in the rest of the tomatoes, cheese, basil, and remaining oil.
- ❖ Thin the mixture with the reserved pasta water if needed.
- ❖ Place in containers and sprinkle with extra cheese.
- ❖ Enjoy!

Nutrition: 340, Total Fat: 11.9 g, Saturated Fat: 3.3 g, Cholesterol: 10 mg, Sodium: 278 mg, Total Carbohydrate: 35.8 g, Dietary Fiber: 7.8 g, Total Sugars: 4.8 g, Protein: 11.6 g, Vitamin D: 0 mcg, Calcium: 193 mg, Iron: 3 mg, Potassium: 524 mg

93) MEDITERRANEAN OLIVE TUNA PASTA

Cooking Time: 20 Minutes **Servings:** 4

Ingredients:

- ✓ 8 ounces of tuna steak, cut into 3 pieces
- ✓ ¼ cup green olives, chopped
- ✓ 3 cloves garlic, minced
- ✓ 2 cups grape tomatoes, halved
- ✓ ½ cup white wine
- ✓ 2 tbsp lemon juice
- ✓ 6 ounces pasta - whole wheat gobetti, rotini, or penne
- ✓ 1 10-ounce package frozen artichoke hearts, thawed and squeezed dry
- ✓ 4 tbsp extra-virgin olive oil, divided
- ✓ 2 tsp fresh grated lemon zest
- ✓ 2 tsp fresh rosemary, chopped, divided
- ✓ ½ tsp salt, divided
- ✓ ¼ tsp fresh ground pepper
- ✓ ¼ cup fresh basil, chopped

Directions:

- ❖ Preheat grill to medium-high heat.
- ❖ Take a large pot of water and put it on to boil.
- ❖ Place the tuna pieces in a bowl and add 1 tbsp of oil, 1 tsp of rosemary, lemon zest, a ¼ tsp of salt, and pepper.
- ❖ Grill the tuna for about 3 minutes per side.
- ❖ Transfer tuna to a plate and allow it to cool.
- ❖ Place the pasta in boiling water and cook according to package instructions.
- ❖ Drain the pasta.
- ❖ Flake the tuna into bite-sized pieces.
- ❖ In a large skillet, heat remaining oil over medium heat.
- ❖ Add artichoke hearts, garlic, olives, and remaining rosemary.
- ❖ Cook for about 3-4 minutes until slightly browned.
- ❖ Add tomatoes, wine, and bring the mixture to a boil.
- ❖ Cook for about 3 minutes until the tomatoes are broken down.
- ❖ Stir in pasta, lemon juice, tuna, and remaining salt.
- ❖ Cook for 1-2 minutes until nicely heated.
- ❖ Spread over the containers.
- ❖ Before eating, garnish with some basil and enjoy!

Nutrition: 455, Total Fat: 21.2 g, Saturated Fat: 3.5 g, Cholesterol: 59 mg, Sodium: 685 mg, Total Carbohydrate: 38.4 g, Dietary Fiber: 6.1 g, Total Sugars: 3.5 g, Protein: 25.5 g, Vitamin D: 0 mcg, Calcium: 100 mg, Iron: 5 mg, Potassium: 800 mg

94) SPECIAL BRAISED ARTICHOKES

Cooking Time: 30 Minutes **Servings:** 6

Ingredients:

- ✓ 6 tbsp olive oil
- ✓ 2 pounds baby artichokes, trimmed
- ✓ ½ cup lemon juice
- ✓ 4 garlic cloves, thinly sliced
- ✓ ½ tsp salt
- ✓ 1½ pounds tomatoes, seeded and diced
- ✓ ½ cup almonds, toasted and sliced

Directions:

- ❖ Heat oil in a skillet over medium heat.
- ❖ Add artichokes, garlic, and lemon juice, and allow the garlic to sizzle.
- ❖ Season with salt.
- ❖ Reduce heat to medium-low, cover, and simmer for about 15 minutes.
- ❖ Uncover, add tomatoes, and simmer for another 10 minutes until the tomato liquid has mostly evaporated.
- ❖ Season with more salt and pepper.
- ❖ Sprinkle with toasted almonds.
- ❖ Enjoy!

Nutrition: Calories: 265, Total Fat: 1g, Saturated Fat: 2.6 g, Cholesterol: 0 mg, Sodium: 265 mg, Total Carbohydrate: 23 g, Dietary Fiber: 8.1 g, Total Sugars: 12.4 g, Protein: 7 g, Vitamin D: 0 mcg, Calcium: 81 mg, Iron: 2 mg, Potassium: 1077 mg

95) DELICIOUS FRIED GREEN BEANS

Cooking Time: 15 Minutes **Servings:** 2

Ingredients:

- ✓ ½ pound green beans, trimmed
- ✓ 1 egg
- ✓ 2 tbsp olive oil
- ✓ 1¼ tbsp almond flour
- ✓ 2 tbsp parmesan cheese
- ✓ ½ tsp garlic powder
- ✓ sea salt or plain salt
- ✓ freshly ground black pepper

Directions:

- ❖ Start by beating the egg and olive oil in a bowl.
- ❖ Then, mix the remaining Ingredients: in a separate bowl and set aside.
- ❖ Now, dip the green beans in the egg mixture and then coat with the dry mix.
- ❖ Finally, grease a baking pan, then transfer the beans to the pan and bake at 5 degrees F for about 12-15 minutes or until crisp.
- ❖ Serve warm.

Nutrition: Calories: 334, Total Fat: 23 g, Saturated Fat: 8.3 g, Cholesterol: 109 mg, Sodium: 397 mg, Total Carbohydrate: 10.9 g, Dietary Fiber: 4.3 g, Total Sugars: 1.9 g, Protein: 18.1 g, Vitamin D: 8 mcg, Calcium: 398 mg, Iron: 2 mg, Potassium: 274 mg

96) VEGGIE MEDITERRANEAN-STYLE PASTA

Cooking Time: 2 Hours   **Servings:** 4

Ingredients:

- 1 tbsp olive oil
- 1 small onion, finely chopped
- 2 small garlic cloves, finely chopped
- 2 14-ounce cans diced tomatoes
- 1 tbsp sun-dried tomato paste
- 1 bay leaf
- 1 tsp dried thyme
- 1 tsp dried basil
- 1 tsp oregano
- 1 tsp dried parsley
- bread of your choice
- ½ tsp salt
- ½ tsp brown sugar
- freshly ground black pepper
- 1 piece aubergine
- 2 pieces courgettes
- 2 pieces red peppers, de-seeded
- 2 garlic cloves, peeled
- 2-3 tbsp olive oil
- 12 small vine-ripened tomatoes
- 16 ounces of pasta of your preferred shape, such as Gigli, conchiglie, etc.
- 3½ ounces parmesan cheese

Directions:

- Heat oil in a pan over medium heat.
- Add onions and fry them until tender.
- Add garlic and stir-fry for 1 minute.
- Add the remaining Ingredients: listed under the sauce and bring to a boil.
- Reduce the heat, cover, and simmer for 60 minutes.
- Season with black pepper and salt as needed. Set aside.
- Preheat oven to 350 degrees F.
- Chop up courgettes, aubergine and red peppers into 1-inch pieces.
- Place them on a roasting pan along with whole garlic cloves.
- Drizzle with olive oil and season with salt and black pepper.
- Mix the veggies well and roast in the oven for 45 minutes until they are tender.
- Add tomatoes just before 20 minutes to end time.
- Cook your pasta according to package instructions.
- Drain well and stir into the sauce.
- Divide the pasta sauce between 4 containers and top with vegetables.
- Grate some parmesan cheese on top and serve with bread.
- Enjoy!

Nutrition: Calories: 211, Total Fat: 14.9 g, Saturated Fat: 2.1 g, Cholesterol: 0 mg, Sodium: 317 mg, Total Carbohydrate: 20.1 g, Dietary Fiber: 5.7 g, Total Sugars: 11.7 g, Protein: 4.2 g, Vitamin D: 0 mcg, Calcium: 66 mg, Iron: 2 mg, Potassium: 955 mg

97) CLASSIC BASIL PASTA

Cooking Time: 40 Minutes   **Servings:** 4

Ingredients:

- 2 red peppers, de-seeded and cut into chunks
- 2 red onions cut into wedges
- 2 mild red chilies, de-seeded and diced
- 3 garlic cloves, coarsely chopped
- 1 tsp golden caster sugar
- 2 tbsp olive oil, plus extra for serving
- 2 pounds small ripe tomatoes, quartered
- 12 ounces pasta
- a handful of basil leaves, torn
- 2 tbsp grated parmesan
- salt
- pepper

Directions:

- Preheat oven to 390 degrees F.
- On a large roasting pan, spread peppers, red onion, garlic, and chilies.
- Sprinkle sugar on top.
- Drizzle olive oil and season with salt and pepper.
- Roast the veggies for 1minutes.
- Add tomatoes and roast for another 15 minutes.
- In a large pot, cook your pasta in salted boiling water according to instructions.
- Once ready, drain pasta.
- Remove the veggies from the oven and carefully add pasta.
- Toss everything well and let it cool.
- Spread over the containers.
- Before eating, place torn basil leaves on top, and sprinkle with parmesan.
- Enjoy!

Nutrition: Calories: 384, Total Fat: 10.8 g, Saturated Fat: 2.3 g, Cholesterol: 67 mg, Sodium: 133 mg, Total Carbohydrate: 59.4 g, Dietary Fiber: 2.3 g, Total Sugars: 5.7 g, Protein: 1 g, Vitamin D: 0 mcg, Calcium: 105 mg, Iron: 4 mg, Potassium: 422 mg

98) ORIGINAL RED ONION KALE PASTA

Cooking Time: 25 Minutes   **Servings: 4**

Ingredients:

- 2½ cups vegetable broth
- ¾ cup dry lentils
- ½ tsp of salt
- 1 bay leaf
- ¼ cup olive oil
- 1 large red onion, chopped
- 1 tsp fresh thyme, chopped
- ½ tsp fresh oregano, chopped
- 1 tsp salt, divided
- ½ tsp black pepper
- 8 ounces vegan sausage, sliced into ¼-inch slices
- 1 bunch kale, stems removed and coarsely chopped
- 1 pack rotini

Directions:

- Add vegetable broth, ½ tsp of salt, bay leaf, and lentils to a saucepan over high heat and bring to a boil.
- Reduce the heat to medium-low and allow to cook for about minutes until tender.
- Discard the bay leaf.
- Take another skillet and heat olive oil over medium-high heat.
- Stir in thyme, onions, oregano, ½ a tsp of salt, and pepper; cook for 1 minute.
- Add sausage and reduce heat to medium-low.
- Cook for 10 minutes until the onions are tender.
- Bring water to a boil in a large pot, and then add rotini pasta and kale.
- Cook for about 8 minutes until al dente.
- Remove a bit of the cooking water and put it to the side.
- Drain the pasta and kale and return to the pot.
- Stir in both the lentils mixture and the onions mixture.
- Add the reserved cooking liquid to add just a bit of moistness.
- Spread over containers.

Nutrition: Calories: 508, Total Fat: 17 g, Saturated Fat: 3 g, Cholesterol: 0 mg, Sodium: 2431 mg, Total Carbohydrate: 59.3 g, Dietary Fiber: 6 g, Total Sugars: 4.8 g, Protein: 30.9 g, Vitamin D: 0 mcg, Calcium: 256 mg, Iron: 8 mg, Potassium: 1686 mg

99) ITALIAN SCALLOPS PEA FETTUCCINE

Cooking Time: 15 Minutes   **Servings: 5**

Ingredients:

- 8 ounces whole-wheat fettuccine (pasta, macaroni)
- 1 pound large sea scallops
- ¼ tsp salt, divided
- 1 tbsp extra virgin olive oil
- 1 8-ounce bottle of clam juice
- 1 cup low-fat milk
- ¼ tsp ground white pepper
- 3 cups frozen peas, thawed
- ¾ cup finely shredded Romano cheese, divided
- 1/3 cup fresh chives, chopped
- ½ tsp freshly grated lemon zest
- 1 tsp lemon juice

Directions:

- Boil water in a large pot and cook fettuccine according to package instructions.
- Drain well and put it to the side.
- Heat oil in a large, non-stick skillet over medium-high heat.
- Pat the scallops dry and sprinkle them with 1/8 tsp of salt.
- Add the scallops to the skillet and cook for about 2-3 minutes per side until golden brown. Remove scallops from pan.
- Add clam juice to the pan you removed the scallops from.
- In another bowl, whisk in milk, white pepper, flour, and remaining 1/8 tsp of salt.
- Once the mixture is smooth, whisk into the pan with the clam juice.
- Bring the entire mix to a simmer and keep stirring for about 1-2 minutes until the sauce is thick.
- Return the scallops to the pan and add peas. Bring it to a simmer.
- Stir in fettuccine, chives, ½ a cup of Romano cheese, lemon zest, and lemon juice.
- Mix well until thoroughly combined.
- Cool and spread over containers.
- Before eating, serve with remaining cheese sprinkled on top.
- Enjoy!

Nutrition: Calories: 388, Total Fat: 9.2 g, Saturated Fat: 3.7 g, Cholesterol: 33 mg, Sodium: 645 mg, Total Carbohydrate: 50.1 g, Dietary Fiber: 10.4 g, Total Sugars: 8.7 g, Protein: 24.9 g, Vitamin D: 25 mcg, Calcium: 293 mg, Iron: 4 mg, Potassium: 247 mg

100) ORIGINAL RED ONION KALE PASTA

Cooking Time: 25 Minutes   **Servings: 4**

Ingredients:

- ✓ 2½ cups vegetable broth
- ✓ ¾ cup dry lentils
- ✓ ½ tsp of salt
- ✓ 1 bay leaf
- ✓ ¼ cup olive oil
- ✓ 1 large red onion, chopped
- ✓ 1 tsp fresh thyme, chopped
- ✓ ½ tsp fresh oregano, chopped
- ✓ 1 tsp salt, divided
- ✓ ½ tsp black pepper
- ✓ 8 ounces vegan sausage, sliced into ¼-inch slices
- ✓ 1 bunch kale, stems removed and coarsely chopped
- ✓ 1 pack rotini

Directions:

- ❖ Add vegetable broth, ½ tsp of salt, bay leaf, and lentils to a saucepan over high heat and bring to a boil.
- ❖ Reduce the heat to medium-low and allow to cook for about minutes until tender.
- ❖ Discard the bay leaf.
- ❖ Take another skillet and heat olive oil over medium-high heat.
- ❖ Stir in thyme, onions, oregano, ½ a tsp of salt, and pepper; cook for 1 minute.
- ❖ Add sausage and reduce heat to medium-low.
- ❖ Cook for 10 minutes until the onions are tender.
- ❖ Bring water to a boil in a large pot, and then add rotini pasta and kale.
- ❖ Cook for about 8 minutes until al dente.
- ❖ Remove a bit of the cooking water and put it to the side.
- ❖ Drain the pasta and kale and return to the pot.
- ❖ Stir in both the lentils mixture and the onions mixture.
- ❖ Add the reserved cooking liquid to add just a bit of moistness.
- ❖ Spread over containers.

Nutrition: Calories: 508, Total Fat: 17 g, Saturated Fat: 3 g, Cholesterol: 0 mg, Sodium: 2431 mg, Total Carbohydrate: 59.3 g, Dietary Fiber: 6 g, Total Sugars: 4.8 g, Protein: 30.9 g, Vitamin D: 0 mcg, Calcium: 256 mg, Iron: 8 mg, Potassium: 1686 mg

101) ITALIAN SCALLOPS PEA FETTUCCINE

Cooking Time: 15 Minutes   **Servings: 5**

Ingredients:

- ✓ 8 ounces whole-wheat fettuccine (pasta, macaroni)
- ✓ 1 pound large sea scallops
- ✓ ¼ tsp salt, divided
- ✓ 1 tbsp extra virgin olive oil
- ✓ 1 8-ounce bottle of clam juice
- ✓ 1 cup low-fat milk
- ✓ ¼ tsp ground white pepper
- ✓ 3 cups frozen peas, thawed
- ✓ ¾ cup finely shredded Romano cheese, divided
- ✓ 1/3 cup fresh chives, chopped
- ✓ ½ tsp freshly grated lemon zest
- ✓ 1 tsp lemon juice

Directions:

- ❖ Boil water in a large pot and cook fettuccine according to package instructions.
- ❖ Drain well and put it to the side.
- ❖ Heat oil in a large, non-stick skillet over medium-high heat.
- ❖ Pat the scallops dry and sprinkle them with 1/8 tsp of salt.
- ❖ Add the scallops to the skillet and cook for about 2-3 minutes per side until golden brown. Remove scallops from pan.
- ❖ Add clam juice to the pan you removed the scallops from.
- ❖ In another bowl, whisk in milk, white pepper, flour, and remaining 1/8 tsp of salt.
- ❖ Once the mixture is smooth, whisk into the pan with the clam juice.
- ❖ Bring the entire mix to a simmer and keep stirring for about 1-2 minutes until the sauce is thick.
- ❖ Return the scallops to the pan and add peas. Bring it to a simmer.
- ❖ Stir in fettuccine, chives, ½ a cup of Romano cheese, lemon zest, and lemon juice.
- ❖ Mix well until thoroughly combined.
- ❖ Cool and spread over containers.
- ❖ Before eating, serve with remaining cheese sprinkled on top.
- ❖ Enjoy!

Nutrition: Calories: 388, Total Fat: 9.2 g, Saturated Fat: 3.7 g, Cholesterol: 33 mg, Sodium: 645 mg, Total Carbohydrate: 50.1 g, Dietary Fiber: 10.4 g, Total Sugars: 8.7 g, Protein: 24.9 g, Vitamin D: 25 mcg, Calcium: 293 mg, Iron: 4 mg, Potassium: 247 mg

PART II: INTRODUCTION

The Mediterranean diet is the most popular and healthy regimen in the world. It is an eating pattern based on the southern European regions' traditional diets surrounding the Mediterranean Sea. Between health benefits, you will reduce the risk of heart disease, diabetes, some types of cancer, and weight problems. This diet is effortless to follow since it is based on whole foods and contains no processed or refined foods. It also promotes a large amount of fiber. The diet focuses on eating lots of fruits, vegetables, whole grains, legumes, nuts, olive oil, and fish. These are all foods that are usually very healthy and delicious, and not too many people have trouble finding them. This book will focus on the main components plus some extra tips that may help you if you are looking to eat for a healthier lifestyle or even live a healthier life in general. Many people say to know the Mediterranean Diet but don't know what it is. If you're new to the Mediterranean Diet or want a guide on how to start eating better, you've come to the right place. Whether you're starting from scratch or already trying to eat healthier, there are several benefits to following this method.

Read these tips and tricks to get started with the Mediterranean Diet today. Many people who have tried the Mediterranean Diet Cookbook have told us that it has made their lives significantly more manageable. So, to help you get started, here's an overview of some of the features and benefits of the Mediterranean Diet. It doesn't take much to save a few calories and a few inches, which is the Mediterranean diet's goal. This comprehensive collection of recipes will show you how to prepare a delicious Mediterranean diet goalie. Remember that there is no particular rule for what you can and cannot eat on a Mediterranean diet. It's all about moderation. Try our recipes and find out if they're right for you!

THE MEDITERRANEAN DIET PYRAMID

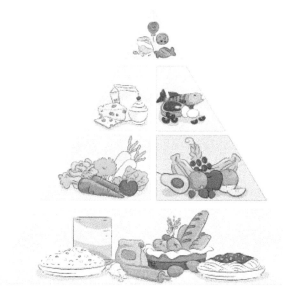

The food pyramid serves as a general guideline on what a healthy, balanced diet should look like. The USDA (United States Department of Agriculture) create this standard scheme so that individuals could follow and better understand the recommended food portions. The USDA food pyramid offered Americans an easy-to-follow template of what they should be eating each day.

This food pyramid well-known version was made public in the 1990s.

At the USDA pyramid base is the grain food group with the recommendation of 6 to 11 servings per day. This group includes bread, pasta, rice, and cereal. Above grains are fruits and vegetables. Fruits recommend 2 to 4 servings per day, while vegetables recommend 3 to 6 servings. The following line on the pyramid is a line that divides the dairy and meat food groups. Dairy products are recommended to be consumed 2 to 3 times a day. The meat group, which includes red meat, poultry, fish, beans, eggs, and nuts, recommends eating 2 to 3 servings per day. At the top of the pyramid, you'll find the "use sparingly" category. In this category, you will find oils, sweets, and fats.

While this pyramid may have helped food manufacturers increase sales, there is a great deal of controversy around it. Not specifying what types of grains should be consumed or healthy and unhealthy fats are the first discrepancies. The other is that the daily recommendations are unbalanced. According to this pyramid, your diet should consist primarily of grains.

The Mediterranean diet pyramid shows that extra virgin olive oil and other healthy fats such as seeds and nuts and whole grains, fruits, vegetables, legumes, and beans are found at the pyramid's base. There are some significant differences between the USDA food pyramid and that of the Mediterranean diet.

First, the USDA has grouped all meat on the pyramid. There is no distinction between whether you should eat more red meat or fish for better overall health.

The Mediterranean diet clearly emphasized fruits, vegetables, and healthy fats to be eaten every day. It also made physical activities and connecting with others a priority. No other diet considered the importance of the latter two factors. While everyone suggests exercise to lose weight, it is rarely indicated as part of a diet plan to live a long healthy life.

It is argued that the Mediterranean diet is not an ideal diet for most people around the world to adapt. As you read on, you'll learn how easy it is to start switching to a Mediterranean diet. You'll see that all of the food groups included in the Mediterranean diet are readily available no matter where you live.

There are so many available diets that people experience great confusion about diets. However, any diet's primary purpose should be to provide a healthy lifestyle, not a bucket list of claims.

One of the best ways to determine which diet will be suitable for your body is to focus on the science behind that diet before following it blindly. Otherwise, he or she will be disappointed if the diet cannot provide the desired results. That's why it's essential to know the complete science behind any diet before following it to save time, energy, resources, and of course, your health.

Most doctors recommend the Mediterranean Diet to patients suffering from heart disease, high blood pressure, depression, or dementia. Let's discuss the science behind this diet to find the reason for its effectiveness.

Most Mediterranean diets differ somewhat from each other. These countries, at that time, showed meager rates of serious diseases, and in those countries, life expectancy was much higher than in other countries of the world. It was believed that the effectiveness of food was due to fresh fruits, vegetables, beans, nuts, grains, fish, olive oil, red wine and cereals, and small amounts of dairy products in Mediterranean kitchens.

The Mediterranean diet is plant-based. This means whole grains, fresh vegetables, fresh fruits, nuts, seeds, herbs, and olive oil, all obtained from plants. Other foods such as animal fats, fish, meat, dairy, and seafood are consumed in smaller amounts. Many studies have shown that this is the best diet globally due to its quick results in achieving a healthy body.

The diet emphasizes healthy fats in olive oil to replace other fats such as butter or margarine. Besides, natural fats in the form of nuts, avocados, fish, etc., contain high amounts of omega-3 fatty acids, essential for a healthy heart.

Also, this diet relies on eating eggs, dairy products, meat, and other animal proteins only once a week or once a month. Eating more vegetables and fruits is why the Mediterranean Diet is more effective than other traditional diets. Another important element of this diet is water as the main drink. Drinking water increases metabolism, promotes a healthy stomach, and improves the digestion system related to weight loss.

Researchers has shown that the Mediterranean Diet is effective against heart disease and provides a healthy body. As mentioned in the study "Mediterranean Diet and Incidence of and Mortality from Coronary Heart Disease and Stroke in Women" by Fung and Rexrode, women who followed the Mediterranean Diet had a 25% lower risk of heart disease and other cardiovascular diseases for almost 12 years.

This diet dispels the myth that eating a low-fat diet helps reduce cardiovascular disease. Eating the correct type of fat is important, not avoiding all fats completely. Studies have shown that the risk factor for heart disease and other chronic diseases is lower when eating the Mediterranean Diet because it replaces bad fats with high-density fats in the form of extra virgin olive oil, nuts, avocados, etc., without ancaloriesie restriction. This diet also reduces the rate of death from stroke. This rate of death reduction is 30% when following the Mediterranean Diet.

Healthy fats from olive oil, fish, avocados, nuts, and seeds makeup 39-42% of your daily caloric intake and are much lighter than consuming any other type of bad fat. The "Reduction in the Incidence of Type 2 Diabetes with the Mediterranean Diet" study showed that this diet reduces the risk of type 2 diabetes.

Another study shows that this diet also helps fight age. As mentioned in the study "The Impact of the Mediterranean Diet on the Cognitive Functioning of Healthy Older Adults: a Systematic Review and Meta-Analysis" by Loughery and Lavecchia, stress and inflammation damage cells. This leads to age-related diseases linked to a specific part of DNA known as "telomeres." These structures shrink with increasing age, causing a shorter life expectancy, so the aging process increases and other age-related diseases. These antioxidants are found in fresh fruits, vegetables, nuts, seeds, whole grains, herbs, and other plant-based products. These foods are significant elements of the Mediterranean Diet. According to the Nurses' Health study, women who followed the Mediterranean Diet had longer telomeres.

In a nutshell, the Mediterranean Diet reduces the risk of chronic disease because it relies on healthy fruits, vegetables, seeds, nuts, herbs, olive oil, grains, and whole grains, which replace foods that contain bad fats. It also contains dairy products, meat, fish, etc., but only once a week or once a month, helping people to have a balanced diet. Besides, the Mediterranean Diet model is a pyramid shape that encourages long-term adherence to the diet foods because it is based on healthy eating and a variety of food, which does not bore a person or negatively affect his mood. Besides, the Mediterranean Diet foods are powerful in fighting several types of diseases, including aging, weight gain, heart problems, stroke, diabetes, inflammation, etc.

THE MEDITERRANEAN DIET: WHAT IS IT?

The term diet often leads you to think you have to count calories, restrict foods and cause a deprivation mentality. A low carb diet, the Atkins diet, the ketogenic diet, and many other diets are formulated to cause rapid weight loss by cutting out nutritional value foods. This is what makes these diets so attractive. While maintaining a healthy weight is an essential aspect of living a healthy life, the focus should not be solely on weight loss.

A diet has to be sustainable. It has to be something that takes a lot of thought and becomes a habit. The Mediterranean diet is not about food restriction. Many people eat without worrying about taking in too many calories. The Mediterranean diet's goal is to help you successfully eliminate the unhealthy foods you consume and replace them with whole foods. It is not just the food and drinks you down, but it also has bits, activities, and people you fill your life.

The Mediterranean diet allows you to live a healthy and fulfilling life. It emphasizes the enjoyment of seasonal and fresh locally grown fruits and vegetables. Food groups such as dairy products and red meat are still valued, but not to the extent that the Western diet tends to products are limited to a few small servings per week, while red meat is included only once or twice a month.

This is not a diet created by research, although it has been thoroughly researched. The Mediterranean diet does not attempt to restrict foods but instead encourages whole, nutritious foods to become a way of life. It is an easy-to-follow way to plan meals inspired by the way people ate in the 1950s and 1960s in the Mediterranean areas. For people who lived there, pre-packaged and processed foods were not readily available. Most people in these areas were not wealthy and grew most of their vegetables and fruits.

You may notice a difference in food choices depending on the region you look. Some areas incorporate more legumes and lentils, while others may enjoy more whole grain options. The similarity, however, is that all of these regions enjoy many plant-based foods and limit or eliminate processed and pre-packaged foods from their diets and added sugars and refined foods. There's not much for people in these areas to think about when it comes to planning their meals. Eating more nutrient-dense foods like fresh fruits and vegetables is such an ingrained way of life for them that they rarely stress about whether they're eating a healthy diet or not.

The Mediterranean diet is inspired by the populations surrounding the Mediterranean Sea. The people of southern Italy and Greece are the central regions that influence this diet. But it is not the diet consumed today in many of these regions that has gained so much attention. The Mediterranean diet refers to the traditional lifestyles of these areas in the 1950s and 1960s. During this time, researchers noticed a significant difference in populations' health in these areas compared to those living in America.

Although it was always evident that the diet of those who resided in Mediterranean regions was healthy, there was little scientific data to link their lifestyle and better health. Ancel Keys was a physiologist who spent much of his career studying dietary patterns and their effects on a person's health. He was a researcher who understood why individuals who lived in the Mediterranean region had much better heart health than those who lived in the United States.

Ancel Keys was incredibly meticulous in his quest to find a connection between diet and heart disease. He believed that saturated fat could be the key culprit that would increase individuals' risk of coronary heart disease. In 1958, he launched what is referred to as the "Seven Country Study" (Rockridge Press, 2013). This study closely examined the eating habits of those residing in Finland, Greece, Italy, Japan, South Africa, Spain, and the United States. Although the data provided by the study included seven countries, 16 cohorts were conducted to participate in the research. There was no financial support to aid the study, which took place over ten years. Each of the countries that agreed to participate in the long-term research did so using their funds, which was a challenge for many countries in the 1960s after the series of wars and struggles most faced.

He found from this study a significantly lower rate of coronary heart disease among even the most impoverished populations in these areas than the population of America. It wasn't just Americans who suffered from increased heart disease. When the American and Finland groups' diets were examined, they found that each consumed a diet high in saturated fat and animal fats.

In contrast, the countries with the lowest heart disease ratios consumed a diet composed primarily of whole grains, fresh vegetables, fish, and unsaturated fats. His findings were among the first to indicate that heart disease and heart attack risk could be prevented.

Despite all the evidence pointing to the Mediterranean diet's undeniable benefits, not everyone is ready to follow the Mediterranean diet. People living today in the Mediterranean do not follow the traditional lifestyle that made the area one of the healthiest worlds just a few decades ago.

There is a debate that much about some of the Mediterranean diet components that distort the facts. This is true for carbohydrates as well. Ancel Keys and many other researchers found that the fats consumed on the Mediterranean diet were very different from the fats consumed in excess in the United States. It was healthy fats such as olive oil that contributed the most to the optimal health of individuals.

Now, a little focus on the red meat issue. Red meat was supposed to be one of the only forms of protein that could be eaten. Eating red meat only occasionally was the opposite of what the U.S. Department of Agriculture was suggesting.

Breakfast

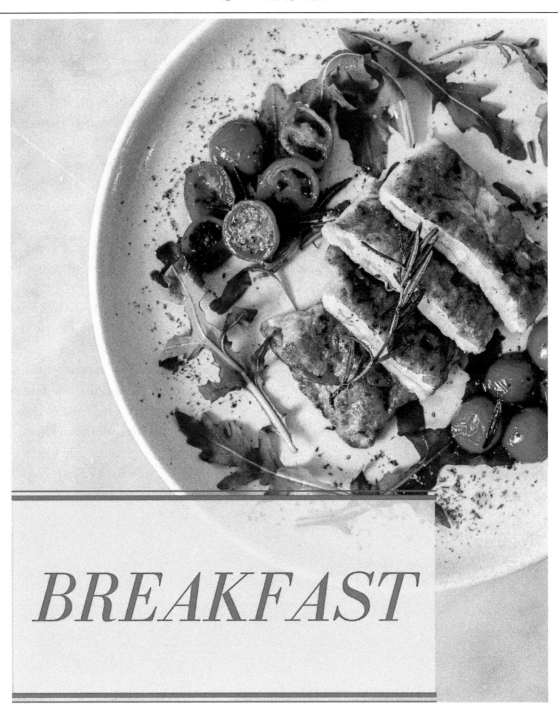

BREAKFAST

102) TAHINI EGG SALAD AND PITA

Cooking Time: 12 Minutes   **Servings: 4**

Ingredients:

- ✓ 4 large eggs
- ✓ ¼ cup freshly chopped dill
- ✓ 1 tbsp plus 1 tsp unsalted tahini
- ✓ 2 tsp freshly squeezed lemon juice
- ✓ ⅛ tsp kosher salt
- ✓ 4 whole-wheat pitas, quartered

Directions:

- ❖ Place the eggs in a saucepan and cover with water. Bring the water to a boil. As soon as the water starts to boil, place a lid on the pan and turn the heat off. Set a timer for minutes.
- ❖ When the timer goes off, drain the hot water and run cold water over the eggs to cool.
- ❖ When the eggs are cool, peel them, place the yolks in a medium bowl, and mash them with a fork. Then chop the egg whites.
- ❖ Add the chopped egg whites, dill, tahini, lemon juice (to taste), and salt to the bowl, and mix to combine.
- ❖ Place a heaping ⅓ cup of egg salad in each of 4 containers. Place the pita in 4 separate containers or resealable bags so that the bread does not get soggy.
- ❖ STORAGE: Store covered containers in the refrigerator for up to 5 days.

Nutrition: Total calories: 242; Total fat: 10g; Saturated fat: 2g; Sodium: 300mg; Carbohydrates: 29g; Fiber: 5g; Protein: 13g

103) MANGO STRAWBERRY- GREEN SMOOTHIE

Cooking Time: 10 Minutes   **Servings: 2**

Ingredients:

- ✓ 1½ cups low-fat (2%) milk
- ✓ 2 cups packed baby spinach leaves
- ✓ ½ cup sliced Persian or English cucumber, skin on
- ✓ ⅔ cup frozen strawberries
- ✓ ⅔ cup frozen mango chunks
- ✓ 1 medium very ripe banana, sliced (about ⅔ cup)
- ✓ ½ small avocado
- ✓ 1 tsp honey

Directions:

- ❖ Place the milk, spinach, cucumber, strawberries, mango, banana, and avocado in a blender.
- ❖ Blend until smooth and taste. If the smoothie isn't sweet enough, add the honey.
- ❖ Distribute the smoothie between 2 to-go cups.
- ❖ STORAGE: Store smoothie cups in the refrigerator for up to 3 days.

Nutrition: Total calories: 261; Total fat: 8g; Saturated fat: 2g; Sodium: 146mg; Carbohydrates: 40g; Fiber: ; Protein: 11g

104) TACO SCRAMBLE BREAKFAST

Cooking Time: 1 Hour 25 Minutes   **Servings: 4**

Ingredients:

- ✓ 8 large eggs, beaten
- ✓ 1/4 tsp seasoning salt
- ✓ 1 lb 99% lean ground turkey
- ✓ 2 tbsp Greek seasoning
- ✓ 1/2 small onion, minced
- ✓ 2 tbsp bell pepper, minced
- ✓ 4 oz. can tomato sauce
- ✓ 1/4 cup water
- ✓ 1/4 cup chopped scallions or cilantro, for topping
- ✓ For the potatoes:
- ✓ 12 (1 lb) baby gold or red potatoes, quartered
- ✓ 4 tsp olive oil
- ✓ 3/4 tsp salt
- ✓ 1/2 tsp garlic powder
- ✓ fresh black pepper, to taste

Directions:

- ❖ In a large bowl, beat the eggs, season with seasoning salt
- ❖ Preheat the oven to 4 degrees F
- ❖ Spray a 9x12 or large oval casserole dish with cooking oil
- ❖ Add the potatoes 1 tbsp oil, 3/tsp salt, garlic powder and black pepper and toss to coat
- ❖ Bake for 4minutes to 1 hour, tossing every 15 minutes
- ❖ In the meantime, brown the turkey in a large skillet over medium heat, breaking it up while it cooks
- ❖ Once no longer pink, add in the Greek seasoning
- ❖ Add in the bell pepper, onion, tomato sauce and water, stir and cover, simmer on low for about 20 minutes
- ❖ Spray a different skillet with nonstick spray over medium heat
- ❖ Once heated, add in the eggs seasoned with 1/4 tsp of salt and scramble for 2–3 minutes, or cook until it sets
- ❖ Distribute 3/4 cup turkey and 2/3 cup eggs and divide the potatoes in each storage container, store for 3-4 days
- ❖ To Serve: Reheat in the microwave for 1-minute (until 90% heated through) top with shredded cheese if desired, and chopped scallions

Nutrition: (¼ of a the scramble): Calories:450;Total Fat: 19g;Total Carbs: 24.5g;Fiber: 4g;Protein: 46g

105)   SPICED PEACH AND ORANGE COMPOTE WITH WHOLE-WHEAT PANCAKES

Cooking Time: 15 Minutes   **Servings:** 6

Ingredients:

- ✓ 1½ cups whole-wheat flour
- ✓ 1 tsp baking powder
- ✓ ½ tsp baking soda
- ✓ ½ tsp ground cinnamon
- ✓ ⅛ tsp kosher salt
- ✓ 1 large egg
- ✓ 1 cup low-fat (2%) plain Greek yogurt
- ✓ 1 tbsp honey
- ✓ 1 cup low-fat (2%) milk
- ✓ 2 tsp olive oil, divided
- ✓ 1 (10-ounce) package frozen sliced peaches
- ✓ ½ cup orange juice
- ✓ ¼ tsp pumpkin pie spice

Directions:

- ❖ TO MAKE THE PANCAKES
- ❖ Combine the flour, baking powder, baking soda, cinnamon, and salt in a large mixing bowl and whisk to make sure everything is distributed evenly. In a separate bowl, whisk together the egg, yogurt, honey, and milk. Pour the liquid ingredients into the dry ingredients and stir until just combined. Do not overmix.
- ❖ Heat ½ tsp of oil in a 12-inch skillet or griddle over medium heat. Once the pan is hot, spoon ¼ cup of pancake batter into the pan. You should be able to fit pancakes in a 12-inch skillet. Cook each side for about 1 minute and 30 seconds, watching carefully and checking the underside for a golden but not burnt color before flipping. Repeat until all the batter has been used.
- ❖ Place 2 pancakes in each of 6 containers.
- ❖ TO MAKE THE COMPOTE
- ❖ Thaw the peaches in the microwave just to the point that they can be cut, about 30 seconds on high. Cut the peaches into 1-inch pieces.
- ❖ Bring the peaches, orange juice, and pumpkin pie spice to a boil in a saucepan. As soon as bubbles appear, lower the heat to medium-low and cook for 12 minutes, until the juice has thickened and the peaches are very soft. Allow to cool, then mash with a potato masher.
- ❖ Place 2 tbsp of compote in each of 6 sauce containers.
- ❖ STORAGE: Store covered pancake containers in the refrigerator for up to 5 days or in the freezer for up to 2 months. Peach compote will last up to 2 weeks in the refrigerator and up to 2 months in the freezer.

Nutrition: Total calories: 209; Total fat: 5g; Saturated fat: 2g; Sodium: 289mg; Carbohydrates: 34g; Fiber: 4g; Protein: 11g

106)   BANANA PEANUT BUTTER GREEK YOGURT

Cooking Time: 5 Minutes   **Servings:** 4

Ingredients:

- ✓ 3 cups vanilla Greek yogurt
- ✓ 2 medium bananas sliced
- ✓ 1/4 cup creamy natural peanut butter
- ✓ 1/4 cup flaxseed meal
- ✓ 1 tsp nutmeg

Directions:

- ❖ Divide yogurt between four jars with lids
- ❖ Top with banana slices
- ❖ In a bowl, melt the peanut butter in a microwave safe bowl for -40 seconds and drizzle one tbsp on each bowl on top of the bananas
- ❖ Store in the fridge for up to 3 days
- ❖ When ready to serve, sprinkle with flaxseed meal and ground nutmeg
- ❖ Enjoy!

Nutrition: Calories:3;Carbs: 47g;Total Fat: 10g;Protein: 22g

107) SHAKSHUKA WITH GREENS

Cooking Time: 15 Minutes   **Servings:** 2

Ingredients:

- ✓ 1 tbsp olive oil
- ✓ 1 onion, peeled and diced
- ✓ 1 clove garlic, peeled and finely minced
- ✓ 3 cups broccoli rabe, chopped
- ✓ 3 cups baby spinach leaves
- ✓ 2 tbsp whole milk or cream
- ✓ 1 tsp ground cumin
- ✓ 1/4 tsp black pepper
- ✓ 1/4 tsp salt (or to taste)
- ✓ 4 Eggs
- ✓ Garnish:
- ✓ 1 pinch sea salt
- ✓ 1 pinch red pepper flakes

Directions:

- ❖ Pre-heat the oven to 350 degrees F
- ❖ Add the broccoli rabe to a large pot of boiling water, cook for minutes, drain and set aside
- ❖ In a large oven-proof skillet or cast-iron pan over medium heat, add in the tbsp of olive oil along with the diced onions, cook for about 10 minutes or until the onions become translucent
- ❖ Add the minced garlic and continue cooking for about another minute
- ❖ Cut the par-cooked broccoli rabe into small pieces, stir into the onion and garlic mixture
- ❖ Cook for a couple of minutes, then stir in the baby spinach leaves, continue to cook for a couple more minutes, stirring often, until the spinach begins to wilt
- ❖ Stir in the ground cumin, salt, ground black pepper, and milk
- ❖ Make four wells in the mixture, crack an egg into each well – be careful not to break the yolks. Also, note that it's easier to crack each egg into a small bowl and then transfer them to the pan
- ❖ Place the pan with the eggs into the pre-heated oven, cook for 10 to 15 minutes until the eggs are set to preference
- ❖ Sprinkle the cooked eggs with a dash of sea salt and a pinch of red pepper flakes
- ❖ Allow to cool, distribute among the containers, store for 2-3 days
- ❖ To Serve: Microwave for 1-minute 0r until heated through, serve with crusty whole-wheat bread or warmed slices of pita or naan

Nutrition: Calories:278; Carbs: 18g;Total Fat: 16g;Protein: 16g

108) TASTY BREAKFAST COOKIES

Cooking Time: 20 Minutes   **Servings:** 4

Ingredients:

- ✓ 2 cups oats (rolled)
- ✓ 1 cup whole wheat flour
- ✓ ¼ cup flax seed
- ✓ 2½ tsp cinnamon (ground)
- ✓ 1 cup honey
- ✓ ½ tsp baking soda
- ✓ 2 egg whites
- ✓ ½ tsp vanilla extract
- ✓ 4 tbsp almond butter
- ✓ pinch of salt

Directions:

- ❖ Preheat oven to 325 degrees F.
- ❖ Whisk oats, flour, flaxseed, cinnamon, salt, and baking soda together in a bowl.
- ❖ Then, stir honey, egg whites, almond butter, and vanilla extract into the oats mixture until dough is blended.
- ❖ Now, prepare the baking sheets and scoop the dough in them.
- ❖ Finally, bake for about 20 minutes.
- ❖ Serve warm or room temperature.

Nutrition: Calories: 686, Total Fat: 14.3g, Saturated Fat: 1.3, Cholesterol: 0 mg, Sodium: 185 mg, Total Carbohydrate: 131.4 g, Dietary Fiber: 11.9 g, Total Sugars: .2 g, Protein: 15.6 g, Vitamin D: 0 mcg, Calcium: 100 mg, Iron: 9 mg, Potassium: 456 mg

109) OMELETTE WITH BROCCOLI AND CHEESE

Cooking Time: 30 Minutes **Servings:** 4

Ingredients:

- ✓ 6 eggs
- ✓ 2 ½ cups of broccoli florets
- ✓ ¼ cup of milk
- ✓ 1 tbsp olive oil
- ✓ ⅓ cup Romano cheese, grated
- ✓ ¼ tsp pepper
- ✓ ⅛ tsp salt
- ✓ ⅓ cup Greek olives, sliced
- ✓ Parsley and more Romano cheese for garnish

Directions:

- ❖ Turn your oven to broil.
- ❖ Set a steamer basket in a large pan and add 1 inch of water.
- ❖ Add the broccoli to the steamer basket and turn the range to medium. Once the water starts to boil, reduce the temperature to low. Steam the broccoli for 4 to 5 minutes. You will know the vegetable is done when it is soft and tender.
- ❖ In a large bowl, whisk the eggs.
- ❖ Pour in the milk, pepper, and salt.
- ❖ Once the broccoli is done, toss into the large bowl and add the olives and grated cheese.
- ❖ Grease an oven-proof 10-inch skillet and turn the heat on the burner to medium.
- ❖ Add in the egg mixture, then cook for 4 to 5 minutes.
- ❖ Set the skillet into the oven but make sure it's at least 4 inches from the heating source. Broil the eggs for 3 minutes. If the eggs are not completely set, continue cooking for another minute or two.
- ❖ Remove the eggs from the oven and set on the stove so they can cool for a few minutes.
- ❖ Garnish the Omelette with cheese and parsley. Then, cut into wedges and enjoy!

Nutrition: calories: 229, fats: 17 grams, carbohydrates: 5 grams, protein: 15 grams.

110) BREAKFAST GREEK YOGURT BOWL

Cooking Time: 5 Minutes **Servings:** 1

Ingredients:

- ✓ 1 cup Greek Yogurt plain
- ✓ 13 cup Pomegranate Seeds (or fresh fruit of your choice)
- ✓ 1 tsp honey

Directions:

- ❖ In a jar with a lid, add the Greek yogurt in a bowl top with fruit and drizzle honey over the top
- ❖ Close the lid and refrigerate for 3 days

Nutrition: Calories116;Carbs 24g;Total Fat 1.2g;Protein 4g

111) CUCUMBER CELERY LIME SMOOTHIE

Cooking Time: 15 Minutes **Servings:** 2

Ingredients:

- ✓ 8 stalks of celery, chopped
- ✓ 1 lemon, juiced
- ✓ 2 cucumbers, peeled and chopped
- ✓ ½ cup ice
- ✓ sweetener of your choice
- ✓ 1 cup water

Directions:

- ❖ Place all the Ingredients: in a blender.
- ❖ Blend well until smooth and frothy or desired texture.
- ❖ Serve chilled.
- ❖ Enjoy.

Nutrition: Calories: 64, Total Fat: 0., Saturated Fat: 0.2, Cholesterol: 0 mg, Sodium: 63 mg, Total Carbohydrate: 15.7 g, Dietary Fiber: 3.4 g, Total Sugars: 6.7 g, Protein: 2.8 g, Vitamin D: 0 mcg, Calcium: 85 mg, Iron: 1 mg, Potassium: 660 mg

112) ALMOND-CHOCOLATE BANANA BREAD

Cooking Time: 25 Minutes   **Servings:** 4

Ingredients:

- ✓ Cooking spray or oil to grease the pan
- ✓ 1 cup almond meal
- ✓ 2 large eggs
- ✓ 2 very ripe bananas, mashed
- ✓ 1 tbsp plus 2 tsp maple syrup
- ✓ ½ tsp vanilla extract
- ✓ ½ tsp baking powder
- ✓ ¼ tsp ground cardamom
- ✓ ⅓ cup dark chocolate chips, very roughly chopped

Directions:

- ❖ Preheat the oven to 350°F and spray an 8-inch cake pan or baking dish with cooking spray or rub with oil.
- ❖ Combine all the ingredients in a large mixing bowl. Then pour the mixture into the prepared pan.
- ❖ Place the pan in the oven and bake for 25 minutes. The edges should be browned, and a paring knife should come out clean when the banana bread is pierced.
- ❖ When cool, slice into wedges and place 1 wedge in each of 4 containers.
- ❖ STORAGE: Store covered containers at room temperature for up to 2 days, refrigerate for up to 7 days, or freeze for up to 3 months.

Nutrition: Total calories: 3; Total fat: 23g; Saturated fat: 6g; Sodium: 105mg; Carbohydrates: 37g; Fiber: 6g; Protein: 10g

113) EGG WHITE SANDWICH MEDITERRANEAN-STYLE BREAKFAST

Cooking Time: 30 Minutes   **Servings:** 1

Ingredients:

- ✓ 1 tsp vegan butter
- ✓ ¼ cup egg whites
- ✓ 1 tsp chopped fresh herbs such as parsley, basil, rosemary
- ✓ 1 whole grain seeded ciabatta roll
- ✓ 1 tbsp pesto
- ✓ 1-2 slices muenster cheese (or other cheese such as provolone, Monterey Jack, etc.)
- ✓ About ½ cup roasted tomatoes
- ✓ Salt, to taste
- ✓ Pepper, to taste
- ✓ Roasted Tomatoes:
- ✓ 10 oz grape tomatoes
- ✓ 1 tbsp extra virgin olive oil
- ✓ Kosher salt, to taste
- ✓ Coarse black pepper, to taste

Directions:

- ❖ In a small nonstick skillet over medium heat, melt the vegan butter
- ❖ Pour in egg whites, season with salt and pepper, sprinkle with fresh herbs, cook for 3-4 minutes or until egg is done, flip once
- ❖ In the meantime, toast the ciabatta bread in toaster
- ❖ Once done, spread both halves with pesto
- ❖ Place the egg on the bottom half of sandwich roll, folding if necessary, top with cheese, add the roasted tomatoes and top half of roll sandwich
- ❖ To make the roasted tomatoes: Preheat oven to 400 degrees F. Slice tomatoes in half lengthwise. Then place them onto a baking sheet and drizzle with the olive oil, toss to coat. Season with salt and pepper and roast in oven for about 20 minutes, until the skin appears wrinkled

Nutrition: Calories:458;Total Carbohydrates: 51g;Total Fat: 0g;Protein: 21g

114) APRICOT-STRAWBERRY SMOOTHIE

Cooking Time: 15 Minutes   **Servings:** 2

Ingredients:

- ✓ 1 cup strawberries, frozen
- ✓ ¾ cup almond milk, unsweetened
- ✓ 2 apricots, pitted and sliced

Directions:

- ❖ Put all the Ingredients: into the blender.
- ❖ Blend them for a minute or until you reach desired foamy texture.
- ❖ Serve the smoothie.
- ❖ Enjoy.

Nutrition: Calories: 247, Total Fat: 21.9 g, Saturated Fat: 19 g, Cholesterol: 0 mg, Sodium: 1mg, Total Carbohydrate: 14.4 g, Dietary Fiber: 4.1 g, Total Sugars: 9.7 g, Protein: 3 g, Vitamin D: 0 mcg, Calcium: 30 mg, Iron: 2 mg, Potassium: 438 mg

115) BREAKFAST BARS WITH APPLE QUINOA

Cooking Time: 40 Minutes   **Servings: 12**

Ingredients:

- ✓ 2 eggs
- ✓ 1 apple peeled and chopped into ½ inch chunks
- ✓ 1 cup unsweetened apple sauce
- ✓ 1 ½ cups cooked & cooled quinoa
- ✓ 1 ½ cups rolled oats
- ✓ 1/4 cup peanut butter
- ✓ 1 tsp vanilla
- ✓ 1/2 tsp cinnamon
- ✓ 1/4 cup coconut oil
- ✓ ½ tsp baking powder

Directions:

- ❖ Heat oven to 350 degrees F
- ❖ Spray an 8x8 inch baking dish with oil, set aside
- ❖ In a large bowl, stir together the apple sauce, cinnamon, coconut oil, peanut butter, vanilla and eggs
- ❖ Add in the cooked quinoa, rolled oats and baking powder, mix until completely incorporated
- ❖ Fold in the apple chunks
- ❖ Spread the mixture into the prepared baking dish, spreading it to each corner
- ❖ Bake for 40 minutes, or until a toothpick comes out clean
- ❖ Allow to cool before slicing
- ❖ Wrap the bars individually in plastic wrap. Store in an airtight container or baggie in the freezer for up to a month.
- ❖ To serve: Warm up in the oven at 350 F for 5 minutes or microwave for up to 30 seconds

Nutrition: (1 bar): Calories:230;Total Fat: 10g;Total Carbs: 31g;Protein: 7g

116) KALE, PEPPER, AND CHICKPEA SHAKSHUKA

Cooking Time: 35 Minutes   **Servings: 5**

Ingredients:

- ✓ 1 tbsp olive oil
- ✓ 1 small red onion, thinly sliced
- ✓ 1 red bell pepper, thinly sliced
- ✓ 1 green bell pepper, thinly sliced
- ✓ 1 bunch kale, stemmed and roughly chopped
- ✓ ½ cup packed cilantro leaves, chopped
- ✓ ½ tsp kosher salt
- ✓ 1 tsp smoked paprika
- ✓ 1 (14.5-ounce) can diced tomatoes
- ✓ 1 (14-ounce) can low-sodium chickpeas, drained and rinsed
- ✓ ⅔ cup water
- ✓ 5 eggs
- ✓ 2½ whole-wheat pitas (optional)

Directions:

- ❖ Preheat the oven to 375°F.
- ❖ Heat the oil in an oven-safe 1inch skillet over medium-high heat. Once the oil is shimmering, add the onions and red and green bell peppers. Sauté for 5 minutes, then cover, leaving the lid slightly ajar. Cook for 5 more minutes, then add the kale and cover, leaving the lid slightly ajar. Cook for 10 more minutes, stirring occasionally.
- ❖ Add the cilantro, salt, paprika, tomatoes, chickpeas, and water, and stir to combine.
- ❖ Make 5 wells in the mixture. Break an egg into a small bowl and pour it into a well. Repeat with the remaining eggs.
- ❖ Place the pan in the oven and bake until the egg whites are opaque and the eggs still jiggle a little when the pan is shaken, about 12 to 1minutes, but start checking at 8 minutes.
- ❖ When the shakshuka is cool, scoop about 1¼ cups of veggies into each of 5 containers, along with 1 egg each. If using, place ½ pita in each of 5 resealable bags.
- ❖ STORAGE: Store covered containers in the refrigerator for up to 5 days.

Nutrition: Total calories: 244; Total fat: 9g; Saturated fat: 2g; Sodium: 529mg; Carbohydrates: 29g; Fiber: ; Protein: 14g

117) BROCCOLI ROSEMARY CAULIFLOWER MASH

Cooking Time: 12 Minutes   **Servings: 3**

Ingredients:

- ✓ 2 cups broccoli, chopped
- ✓ 1 lb cauliflower, cut into florets
- ✓ 1 tsp dried rosemary
- ✓ 1/4 cup olive oil
- ✓ 1 tsp garlic, minced
- ✓ Salt

Directions:

- ❖ Add broccoli and cauliflower into the instant pot. Pour enough water into the pot to cover broccoli and cauliflower.
- ❖ Seal pot with lid and cook on high for 1minutes.
- ❖ Once done, allow to release pressure naturally. Remove lid.
- ❖ Drain broccoli and cauliflower well and clean the instant pot.
- ❖ Add oil into the pot and set the pot on sauté mode.
- ❖ Add broccoli, cauliflower, rosemary, garlic, and salt and cook for 10 minutes.
- ❖ Mash the broccoli and cauliflower mixture using a potato masher until smooth.
- ❖ Serve and enjoy.

Nutrition: Calories: 205;Fat: 17.2 g;Carbohydrates: 12.6 g;Sugar: 4.7 g;Protein: 4.8 g;Cholesterol: 0 mg

118) APPLE, PUMPKIN, AND GREEK YOGURT MUFFINS

Cooking Time: 20 Minutes   **Servings: 12**

Ingredients:

- ✓ Cooking spray to grease baking liners
- ✓ 2 cups whole-wheat flour
- ✓ 1 tsp aluminum-free baking powder (see tip)
- ✓ 1 tsp baking soda
- ✓ ⅛ tsp kosher salt
- ✓ 2 tsp ground cinnamon
- ✓ ½ tsp ground ginger
- ✓ ½ tsp ground allspice
- ✓ ⅔ cup pure maple syrup
- ✓ 1 cup low-fat (2%) plain Greek yogurt
- ✓ 1 cup 100% canned pumpkin
- ✓ 1 large egg
- ✓ ¼ cup extra-virgin olive oil
- ✓ 1½ cups chopped green apple (leave peel on)
- ✓ ½ cup walnut pieces

Directions:

- ❖ Preheat the oven to 400°F and line a muffin tin with baking liners. Spray the liners lightly with cooking spray.
- ❖ In a large bowl, whisk together the flour, baking powder, baking soda, salt, cinnamon, ginger, and allspice.
- ❖ In a medium bowl, combine the maple syrup, yogurt, pumpkin, egg, olive oil, chopped apple, and walnuts.
- ❖ Pour the wet ingredients into the dry ingredients and combine just until blended. Do not overmix.
- ❖ Scoop about ¼ cup of batter into each muffin liner and bake for 20 minutes, or until the tops look browned and a paring knife comes out clean when inserted. Remove the muffins from the tin to cool.
- ❖ STORAGE: Store covered containers at room temperature for up to 4 days. To freeze the muffins for up to 3 months, wrap them in foil and place in an airtight resealable bag.

Nutrition: Total calories: 221; Total fat: 9g; Saturated fat: 1g; Sodium: 18g; Carbohydrates: 32g; Fiber: 4g; Protein: 6g

119) COCOA WITH RASPBERRY OVERNIGHT OATS

Cooking Time: 10 Minutes   **Servings: 5**

Ingredients:

- ✓ 1⅔ cups rolled oats
- ✓ 3⅓ cups unsweetened vanilla almond milk
- ✓ 2 tsp vanilla extract
- ✓ 1 tbsp plus 2 tsp pure maple syrup
- ✓ 3 tbsp chia seeds
- ✓ 3 tbsp unsweetened cocoa powder
- ✓ 1⅔ cups frozen raspberries
- ✓ 5 tsp cocoa nibs (optional)

Directions:

- ❖ In a large bowl, mix the oats, almond milk, vanilla, maple syrup, chia seeds, and cocoa powder until well combined.
- ❖ Spoon ¾ cup of the oat mixture into each of 5 containers.
- ❖ Top each serving with ⅓ cup of raspberries and 1 tsp of cocoa nibs, if using.
- ❖ STORAGE: Store covered containers in the refrigerator for up to 5 days.

Nutrition: Total calories: 21 Total fat: 6g; Saturated fat: <1g; Sodium: 121mg; Carbohydrates: 34g; Fiber: 10g; Protein: 7g

120) BACON BRIE OMELETTE WITH RADISH SALAD

Cooking Time: 10 Minutes   **Servings: 6**

Ingredients:

- 200 g smoked lardons
- 3 tsp olive oil, divided
- 7 ounces smoked bacon
- 6 lightly beaten eggs
- small bunch chives, snipped up

- 3½ ounces sliced brie
- 1 tsp red wine vinegar
- 1 tsp Dijon mustard
- 1 cucumber, deseeded, halved, and sliced up diagonally
- 7 ounces radish, quartered

Directions:

- Heat up the grill.
- Add 1 tsp of oil to a small pan and heat on the grill.
- Add lardons and fry them until nice and crisp.
- Drain the lardon on kitchen paper.
- Heat the remaining 2 tsp of oil in a non-sticking pan on the grill.
- Add lardons, eggs, chives, and ground pepper, and cook over low heat until semi-set.
- Carefully lay the Brie on top, and grill until it has set and is golden in color.
- Remove from pan and cut into wedges.
- Make the salad by mixing olive oil, mustard, vinegar, and seasoning in a bowl.
- Add cucumber and radish and mix well.
- Serve the salad alongside the Omelette wedges in containers.
- Enjoy!

Nutrition: Calories: 620, Total Fat: 49.3g, Saturated Fat: 22.1, Cholesterol: 295 mg, Sodium: 1632 mg, Total Carbohydrate: 4.3g, Dietary Fiber: 0.9 g, Total Sugars: 2.5 g, Protein: 39.2 g, Vitamin D: 41 mcg, Calcium: 185 mg, Iron: 2 mg, Potassium: 527 mg

121) OATMEAL WITH CRANBERRIES

Cooking Time: 6 Minutes   **Servings: 2**

Ingredients:

- 1/2 cup steel-cut oats
- 1 cup unsweetened almond milk
- 1 1/2 tbsp maple syrup
- 1/4 tsp cinnamon

- 1/4 tsp vanilla
- 1/4 cup dried cranberries
- 1 cup of water
- 1 tsp lemon zest, grated
- 1/4 cup orange juice

Directions:

- Add all ingredients into the heat-safe dish and stir well.
- Pour 1 cup of water into the instant pot then place the trivet in the pot.
- Place dish on top of the trivet.
- Seal pot with lid and cook on high for 6 minutes.
- Once done, allow to release pressure naturally for 10 minutes then release remaining using quick release. Remove lid.
- Serve and enjoy.

Nutrition: Calories: 161;Fat: 3.2 g;Carbohydrates: 29.9 g;Sugar: 12.4 g;Protein: 3.4 g;Cholesterol: 0 mg

122) FIG TOAST WITH RICOTTA

Cooking Time: 15 Minutes   **Servings: 1**

Ingredients:

- 2 slices whole-wheat toast
- 1 tsp honey
- ¼ cup ricotta (partly skimmed)

- 1 dash cinnamon
- 2 figs (sliced)
- 1 tsp sesame seeds

Directions:

- Start by mixing ricotta with honey and dash of cinnamon.
- Then, spread this mixture on the toast.
- Now, top with fig and sesame seeds.
- Serve.

Nutrition: Calories: 372, Total Fat: 8.8g, Saturated Fat: 3.8, Cholesterol: 19 mg, Sodium: 373 mg, Total Carbohydrate: .7 g, Dietary Fiber: 8.8 g, Total Sugars: 27.1 g, Protein: 17 g, Vitamin D: 0 mcg, Calcium: 328 mg, Iron: 3 mg, Potassium: 518 mg

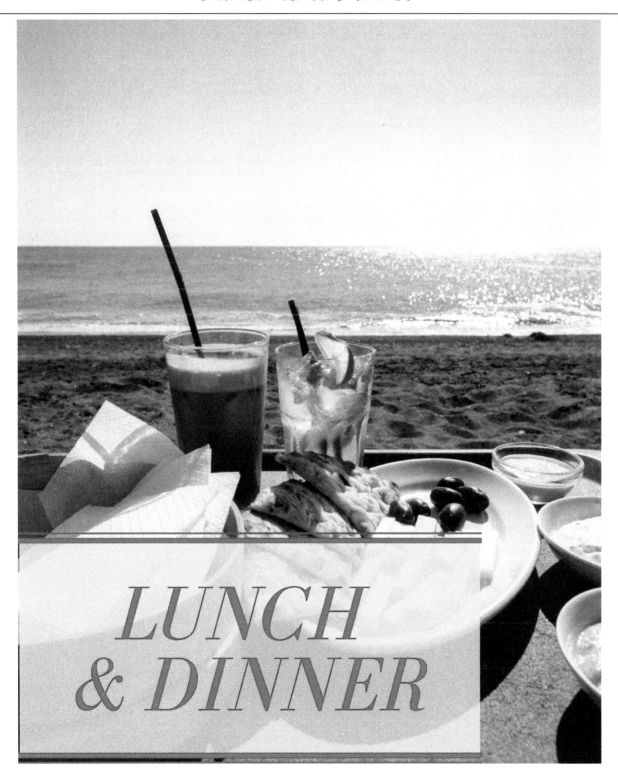

LUNCH & DINNER

123) CARROT SOUP AND PARMESAN CROUTONS

Cooking Time: 25 To 30 Minutes   **Servings: 4**

Ingredients:

- ✓ 2 cups vegetable broth, no salt added, and low sodium is best
- ✓ 1 tsp dried thyme
- ✓ ¼ tsp sea salt
- ✓ 1 ounce grated parmesan cheese
- ✓ 2 pounds of carrots, unpeeled
- ✓ 2 tbsp extra virgin olive oil
- ✓ ½ chopped onion
- ✓ 2 ½ cups water
- ✓ ¼ tsp crushed red pepper
- ✓ 4 slices of whole-grain bread

Directions:

- ❖ Cut your carrots into ½-inch slices
- ❖ Take one rack from your oven and place it four inches from the broiler heating element. One either rack, place two large-rimmed baking sheets and turn your oven to 450 degrees Fahrenheit.
- ❖ Add 1 tbsp of oil and carrots into a large bowl. Stir the carrots around so they become coated with the oil.
- ❖ Using oven mitts, remove the baking pans and distribute the carrots onto them.
- ❖ Place the pans back into the oven and turn your timer on for 20 minutes or until the carrots become tender.
- ❖ Take the carrots out of the oven.
- ❖ Turn your oven to broiler mode.
- ❖ Set a large stockpot on your stove and turn the range to medium-high.
- ❖ Pour in the remaining olive oil and the onion. Let it cook for 5 minutes while stirring occasionally.
- ❖ Pour in the broth, thyme, water, crushed red pepper, and sea salt. Stir well.
- ❖ Let the mixture cook until the ingredients come to a boil.
- ❖ Once the carrots are done in the oven, add them to the pot.
- ❖ Remove the pot from the heat and carefully pour the soup into a blender. You will want to pour it in batches and remember to hold the lid of the blender with a rag and release the steam after 30 seconds, so it doesn't explode.
- ❖ Once all the soup is mixed, add it all back into the pot and turn the range heat to medium. Cook until the soup is warm again.
- ❖ Spread a piece of parchment paper on top of a baking sheet, set the four pieces of bread on the paper.
- ❖ Sprinkle cheese across the slices and set them on the top rack in your oven.
- ❖ Turn your oven to broil and let the slices of bread roast for a couple of minutes. Once the cheese is melted, remove the bread from the oven so they don't burn.
- ❖ Chop the bread into croutons.
- ❖ Divide the soup into serving bowls, add the croutons, and enjoy!

Nutrition: Nutrition: calories: 272, fats: 10 grams, carbohydrates: 38 grams, protein: 10 grams.

124) GREEK-STYLE BAKED COD

Cooking Time: 12 Minutes   **Servings:** 4

Ingredients:

- 1 ½ lb Cod fillet pieces (4–6 pieces)
- 5 garlic cloves, peeled and minced
- 1/4 cup chopped fresh parsley leaves
- Lemon Juice Mixture:
- 5 tbsp fresh lemon juice
- 5 tbsp extra virgin olive oil
- 2 tbsp melted vegan butter
- For Coating:
- 1/3 cup all-purpose flour
- 1 tsp ground coriander
- 3/4 tsp sweet Spanish paprika
- 3/4 tsp ground cumin
- 3/4 tsp salt
- 1/2 tsp black pepper

Directions:

- Preheat oven to 400 degrees F
- In a bowl, mix together lemon juice, olive oil, and melted butter, set aside
- In another shallow bowl, mix all-purpose flour, spices, salt and pepper, set next to the lemon bowl to create a station
- Pat the fish fillet dry, then dip the fish in the lemon juice mixture then dip it in the flour mixture, shake off excess flour
- In a cast iron skillet over medium-high heat, add 2 tbsp olive oil
- Once heated, add in the fish and sear on each side for color, but do not fully cook (just couple minutes on each side), remove from heat
- With the remaining lemon juice mixture, add the minced garlic and mix
- Drizzle all over the fish fillets
- Bake for 10 minutes, for until the it begins to flake easily with a fork
- allow the dish to cool completely
- Distribute among the containers, store for 2-3 days
- To Serve: Reheat in the microwave for 1-2 minutes or until heated through. Sprinkle chopped parsley. Enjoy!

Nutrition: Calories:321;Carbs: 16g;Total Fat: 18g;Protein: 23g

125) SOLE FISH WITH PISTACHIO

Cooking Time: 10 Minutes   **Servings:** 4

Ingredients:

- 4 (5 ounces boneless sole fillets
- Salt and pepper as needed
- ½ cup pistachios, finely chopped
- Zest of 1 lemon
- Juice of 1 lemon
- 1 tsp extra virgin olive oil

Directions:

- Pre-heat your oven to 350 degrees Fahrenheit
- Line a baking sheet with parchment paper and keep it on the side
- Pat fish dry with kitchen towels and lightly season with salt and pepper
- Take a small bowl and stir in pistachios and lemon zest
- Place sol on the prepped sheet and press 2 tbsp of pistachio mixture on top of each fillet
- Drizzle fish with lemon juice and olive oil
- Bake for 10 minutes until the top is golden and fish flakes with a fork
- Serve and enjoy!
- Meal Prep/Storage Options: Store in airtight containers in your fridge for 1-2 days.

Nutrition: Calories: 166;Fat: 6g;Carbohydrates: 2g;Protein: 26g

126)   TOMATO SOUP WITH BEEF

Cooking Time: 1 Hour   **Servings: 6**

Ingredients:

- ✓ 1 pound lean ground beef
- ✓ 1 medium onion, chopped
- ✓ 1 large green pepper, chopped
- ✓ 2 minced garlic cloves
- ✓ 1 large tomato, chopped
- ✓ 2 tbsp tomato paste
- ✓ 2 tbsp all-purpose flour
- ✓ ¼ cup uncooked rice
- ✓ 2 tbsp fresh chopped parsley (additional for garnish)
- ✓ 4 cups beef broth
- ✓ 2 tbsp olive oil
- ✓ salt
- ✓ pepper

Directions:

- ❖ Add oil to large pot and heat over medium heat.
- ❖ Add flour and keep whisking until thick paste forms.
- ❖ Keep whisking for 4 minutes while it bubbles and begins to thin.
- ❖ Add onions and sauté for 3-minutes.
- ❖ Stir in tomato paste and ground beef, breaking up ground beef with a wooden spoon.
- ❖ Cook for about 5 minutes.
- ❖ Add garlic, peppers, and tomatoes.
- ❖ Mix well until thoroughly combined.
- ❖ Add broth and bring the mixture to a light boil.
- ❖ Reduce heat to low, cover, and simmer for 30 minutes, making sure to stir from time to time.
- ❖ Add rice and parsley and cook for another 15 minutes.
- ❖ Once the soup has achieved its desired consistency, serve with a garnish of parsley.
- ❖ This soup is best enjoyed with some crispy bread or boiled potatoes.

Nutrition: Calories: 268, Total Fat: 10.6 g, Saturated Fat: 2.8 g, Cholesterol: 68 mg, Sodium: 568 mg, Total Carbohydrate: 3 g, Dietary Fiber: 1.7 g, Total Sugars: 3.4 g, Protein: 28 g, Vitamin D: 0 mcg, Calcium: 25 mg, Iron: 15 mg, Potassium: 665 mg

127)   BAKED TILAPIA

Cooking Time: 15 Minutes   **Servings: 4**

Ingredients:

- ✓ 1 lb tilapia fillets (about 8 fillets)
- ✓ 1 tsp olive oil
- ✓ 1 tbsp vegan butter
- ✓ 2 shallots finely chopped
- ✓ 3 garlic cloves minced
- ✓ 1 1/2 tsp ground cumin
- ✓ 1 1/2 tsp paprika
- ✓ 1/4 cup capers
- ✓ 1/4 cup fresh dill finely chopped
- ✓ Juice from 1 lemon
- ✓ Salt & Pepper to taste

Directions:

- ❖ Preheat oven to 375 degrees F
- ❖ Line a rimmed baking sheet with parchment paper or foil
- ❖ Lightly mist with cooking spray, arrange the fish fillets evenly on baking sheet
- ❖ In a small bowl, combine the cumin, paprika, salt and pepper
- ❖ Season both sides of the fish fillets with the spice mixture
- ❖ In a small bowl, whisk together the melted butter, lemon juice, shallots, olive oil, and garlic, and brush evenly over fish fillets
- ❖ Top with the capers
- ❖ Bake in the oven for 10-15 minutes, until cook through, but not overcooked
- ❖ Remove from oven and allow the dish to cool completely
- ❖ Distribute among the containers, store for 2-3 days
- ❖ To Serve: Reheat in the microwave for 1-2 minutes or until heated through. Top with fresh dill. Serve!

Nutrition: Calories:;Total Fat: 5g;Protein: 21g

128) HERBAL LAMB CUTLETS AND ROASTED VEGGIES

Cooking Time: 45 Minutes   **Servings:** 6

Ingredients:

- 2 deseeded peppers, cut up into chunks
- 1 large sweet potato, peeled and chopped
- 2 sliced courgettes
- 1 red onion, cut into wedges
- 1 tbsp olive oil
- 8 lean lamb cutlets
- 1 tbsp thyme leaf, chopped
- 2 tbsp mint leaves, chopped

Directions:

- Preheat oven to 390degrees F.
- In a large baking dish, place peppers, courgettes, sweet potatoes, and onion.
- Drizzle all with oil and season with ground pepper.
- Roast for about 25 minutes
- Trim as much fat off the lamb as possible.
- Mix in herbs with a few twists of ground black pepper.
- Take the veggies out of the oven and push to one side of a baking dish.
- Place lamb cutlets on another side, return to oven, and roast for another 10 minutes.
- Turn the cutlets over, cook for another 10 minutes, and until the veggies are ready (lightly charred and tender).
- Mix everything on the tray and spread over containers.

Nutrition: Calories: 268, Total Fat: 9.2 g, Saturated Fat: 3 g, Cholesterol: 100 mg, Sodium: mg, Total Carbohydrate: 10.7 g, Dietary Fiber: 2.4 g, Total Sugars: 4.1 g, Protein: 32.4 g, Vitamin D: 0 mcg, Calcium: 20 mg, Iron: 4 mg, Potassium: 365 mg

129) WONDERFUL MEDITERRANEAN-STYLE SNAPPER

Cooking Time: 10 Minutes   **Servings:** 2

Ingredients:

- 2 tbsp extra virgin olive oil
- 1 medium onion, chopped
- 2 garlic cloves, minced
- 1 tsp oregano
- 1 can (14 ounces tomatoes, diced with juice
- ½ cup black olives, sliced
- 4 red snapper fillets (each 4 ounce
- Salt and pepper as needed
- Garnish
- ¼ cup feta cheese, crumbled
- ¼ cup parsley, minced

Directions:

- Pre-heat your oven to a temperature of 425-degree Fahrenheit
- Take a 13x9 inch baking dish and grease it up with non-stick cooking spray
- Take a large sized skillet and place it over medium heat
- Add oil and heat it up
- Add onion, oregano and garlic
- Saute for 2 minutes
- Add diced tomatoes with juice alongside black olives
- Bring the mix to a boil
- Remove the heat
- Place the fish on the prepped baking dish
- Season both sides with salt and pepper
- Spoon the tomato mix over the fish
- Bake for 10 minutes
- Remove the oven and sprinkle a bit of parsley and feta
- Enjoy!
- Meal Prep/Storage Options: Store in airtight containers in your fridge for 1-3 days

Nutrition: Calories: 269;Fat: 13g;Carbohydrates: 10g;Protein: 27g

130) MEDITERRANEAN-STYLE SNAPPER

Cooking Time: 12 Minutes   **Servings: 4**

Ingredients:

- ✓ non-stick cooking spray
- ✓ 2 tbsp extra virgin olive oil
- ✓ 1 medium onion, chopped
- ✓ 2 garlic cloves, minced
- ✓ 1 tsp oregano
- ✓ 1 14-ounce can diced tomatoes, undrained

- ✓ ½ cup black olives, sliced
- ✓ 4 4-ounce red snapper fillets
- ✓ salt
- ✓ pepper
- ✓ ¼ cup crumbled feta cheese
- ✓ ¼ cup fresh parsley, minced

Directions:

- ❖ Preheat oven to 425 degrees Fahrenheit.
- ❖ Grease a 13x9 baking dish with non-stick cooking spray.
- ❖ Heat oil in a large skillet over medium heat.
- ❖ Add onion, oregano, garlic, and sauté for 2 minutes.
- ❖ Add can of tomatoes and olives, and bring mixture to a boil; remove from heat.
- ❖ Season both sides of fillets with salt and pepper and place in the baking dish.
- ❖ Spoon the tomato mixture evenly over the fish.
- ❖ Bake for 10 minutes.
- ❖ Remove from oven and sprinkle with parsley and feta.
- ❖ Enjoy!

Nutrition: Calories: 257, Total Fat: g, Saturated Fat: 1.7 g, Cholesterol: 53 mg, Sodium: 217 mg, Total Carbohydrate: 8.2 g, Dietary Fiber: 2.5 g, Total Sugars: 3.8 g, Protein: 31.3 g, Vitamin D: 0 mcg, Calcium: 85 mg, Iron: 1 mg, Potassium: 881 mg

131) ITALIAN SKILLET CHICKEN AND MUSHROOMS WITH TOMATOES

Cooking Time: 20 Minutes   **Servings: 4**

Ingredients:

- ✓ 4 large chicken cutlets, boneless skinless chicken breasts cut into 1/4-inch thin cutlets
- ✓ 1 tbsp dried oregano, divided
- ✓ 1/2 cup all-purpose flour, more for later
- ✓ 8 oz Baby Bella mushrooms, cleaned, trimmed, and sliced
- ✓ 14 oz grape tomatoes, halved
- ✓ 2 tbsp chopped fresh garlic

- ✓ Extra Virgin Olive Oil
- ✓ 1/2 cup white wine
- ✓ 1 tbsp freshly squeezed lemon juice, juice of 1/2 lemon
- ✓ 1 tsp salt, divided
- ✓ 1 tsp black pepper, divided
- ✓ 3/4 cup chicken broth
- ✓ Handful baby spinach, optional

Directions:

- ❖ Pat the chicken cutlets dry, season both sides with 2 tsp salt, 1/2 tsp black pepper, 1/2 tbsp dried oregano,
- ❖ Coat the chicken cutlets with the flour, gently dust-off excess and set aside
- ❖ In a large cast iron skillet with a lid, heat 2 tbsp olive oil
- ❖ Once heated, brown the chicken cutlets on both sides, for about 3 minutes, then transfer the chicken cutlets to plate
- ❖ In the same skillet, add more olive oil if needed,
- ❖ Once heated, add in the mushrooms and sauté on medium-high for about 1 minute
- ❖ Then add the tomatoes, garlic, the remaining 1/2 tbsp oregano, 1/2 tsp salt, and 1/2 tsp pepper, and 2 tsp flour, cook for 3 minutes or so, stirring regularly
- ❖ Add in the white wine, cook briefly to reduce, then add the lemon juice and chicken broth
- ❖ Bring the liquid to a boil, then transfer the chicken back into the skillet, cook over high heat for 3-4 minutes, then reduce the heat to medium-low, cover and cook for another 8 minutes or until the chicken is cooked through
- ❖ Allow the dish to cool completely
- ❖ Distribute among the containers, store for 3 days
- ❖ To Serve: Reheat in the microwave for 1-2 minutes or until heated through. Serve with baby spinach, your favorite small pasta and a crusty Italian bread!

Nutrition: Calories:218;Carbs: 16g;Total Fat: 6g;Protein: 23g

132) RED WINE–BRAISED POT ROAST AND CARROTS WITH MUSHROOMS

Cooking Time: 25 Minutes   **Servings: 4**

Ingredients:

- 1 pound tri-tip roast
- ¼ tsp kosher salt
- 1 tbsp olive oil
- 2 cups chopped onion
- 1 tsp chopped garlic
- 3 medium carrots, cut into ½-inch pieces (2 cups)
- 2 large celery stalks, cut into ½-inch pieces (1 cup)
- 8 ounces button or cremini mushrooms, halved
- ½ tsp fennel seed
- ½ tsp dried thyme
- ½ tsp dried oregano
- 1 (14.5-ounce) can no-salt-added diced tomatoes
- 1 cup dry red wine, such as red zinfandel or cabernet sauvignon
- 1 cup reduced-sodium beef broth

Directions:

- Preheat the oven to 325°F.
- Season the roast with the salt.
- Heat the oil in a Dutch oven or heavy-bottomed soup pot over high heat. Once the oil is hot, add the roast and brown for minutes on each side. Remove the roast to a plate.
- Add the onion, garlic, carrots, celery, and mushrooms to the pot and cook for 5 minutes.
- Add the fennel seed, thyme, oregano, tomatoes, red wine, and broth and bring to a simmer. Cover the pot with a tight-fitting lid or foil and place in the oven. Cook until the meat is very tender, about 3 hours.
- Remove the roast to a plate and spoon the vegetables into a bowl with a slotted spoon. Place the pot on high heat and reduce the liquid by half, about 10 minutes. If your pot is extra wide, it will take less time for the liquid to reduce. Add more salt if needed.
- After the meat has cooled, cut 12 slices against the grain. Place 3 slices, ¾ cup of vegetables, and ⅓ cup of sauce in each of 4 containers.
- STORAGE: Store covered containers in the refrigerator for up to 5 days.

Nutrition: Total calories: 366; Total fat: 14g; Saturated fat: 4g; Sodium: 468mg; Carbohydrates: 23g; Fiber: 6g; Protein: 28g

133) ZOODLES AND TURKEY MEATBALLS

Cooking Time: 30 Minutes   **Servings: 4-6**

Ingredients:

- 2 lbs (3 medium-sized) zucchini, spiralized
- 2 cups marinara sauce, store-bought
- 1/4 cup freshly grated Parmesan cheese
- 2 tsp salt
- For The Meatballs:
- 1 ½ lbs ground turkey
- 1/2 cup Panko
- 1/4 cup freshly grated Parmesan cheese
- 2 large egg yolks
- 1 tsp dried oregano
- 1 tsp dried basil
- 1/2 tsp dried parsley
- 1/4 tsp garlic powder
- 1/4 tsp crushed red pepper flakes
- Kosher salt, to taste
- Freshly ground black pepper, to taste

Directions:

- Preheat oven to 400 degrees F
- Lightly oil a 9×13 baking dish or spray with nonstick spray
- In a large bowl, combine the ground turkey, egg yolks, oregano, basil, Panko, Parmesan, parsley, garlic powder and red pepper flakes, season the mixture with salt and pepper, to taste
- Use a wooden spoon or clean hands, stir well to combined
- Roll the mixture into 1 1/2-to-2-inch meatballs, forming about 24 meatballs
- Place the meatballs onto the prepared baking dish
- Bake for 18-20 minutes, or until browned and the meatballs are cooked through, set aside
- Place the zucchini in a colander over the sink, add the salt and gently toss to combine, allow to sit for 10 minutes
- In a large pot of boiling water, cook zucchini for 30 seconds to 1 minute, drain well
- Allow to cool, then distribute the zucchini into the containers, top with the meatballs, marinara sauce and the Parmesan. Store in the fridge for up to 4 days
- To Serve: Reheat in the microwave for 1-2 minutes or until heated through and enjoy!

Nutrition: Calories:279;Total Fat: 13g;Total Carbs: ;Fiber: 3g;Protein: 31g

134)   ITALIAN PLATTER

Cooking Time: 45 Minutes   **Servings: 2**

Ingredients:

- 1 garlic clove, minced
- 5-ounce fresh button mushrooms, sliced
- 1/8 cup unsalted butter
- ¼ tsp dried thyme
- 1/3 cup heavy whipping cream
- Salt and black pepper, to taste
- 2 (6-ounce grass-fed New York strip steaks

Directions:

- Preheat the grill to medium heat and grease it.
- Season the steaks with salt and black pepper, and transfer to the grill.
- Grill steaks for about 10 minutes on each side and dish out in a platter.
- Put butter, mushrooms, salt and black pepper in a pan and cook for about 10 minutes.
- Add thyme and garlic and thyme and sauté for about 1 minute.
- Stir in the cream and let it simmer for about 5 minutes.
- Top the steaks with mushroom sauce and serve hot immediately.
- Meal Prep Tip: You can store the mushroom sauce in refrigerator for about 2 days. Season the steaks carefully with salt and black pepper to avoid low or high quantities.

Nutrition: Calories: 332 ;Carbohydrates: 3.2g;Protein: 41.8g;Fat: 20.5g ;Sugar: 1.3g;Sodium: 181mg

135)   MEDITERRANEAN-STYLE PIZZA

Cooking Time: 20 Minutes   **Servings: 4 To 8**

Ingredients:

- 1/2 cup artichoke hearts
- Whole-wheat premade pizza crust
- 1 cup pesto sauce
- 1 cup spinach leaves
- 3 to 4 ounces of feta cheese
- 1 cup sun-dried tomatoes
- 3 ounces of mozzarella cheese
- ½ cup of olives
- Olive oil
- ½ cup bell peppers
- Chopped chicken, pepperoni, or salami

Directions:

- Turn the temperature of your oven to 350 degrees Fahrenheit.
- Use olive oil to brush the top of the whole wheat pizza crust.
- Brush the pesto sauce on the pizza crust.
- Top with all of the ingredients. You can start with the cheese or mix the ingredients in any way you wish. You can even get a little creative and have fun.
- Set your pizza on a pizza pan or directly on your oven rack.
- Set your timer to 10 minutes, but watch the pizza carefully so you do not burn the cheese.
- Remove the pizza and let it cool down for a couple of minutes, then enjoy!

Nutrition: calories: 300, fats: 11 grams, carbohydrates: 29 grams, protein: 14 grams.

136) VEGETABLE QUINOA BOWL ROAST

Cooking Time: 20 Minutes   **Servings: 2**

Ingredients:

- Quinoa:
- ¾ cup quinoa, rinsed
- 1 ½ cups
- vegetable broth
- Chili-Lime Kale
- 1/2 tsp chili powder
- pinch salt
- pinch pepper
- 2 cups packed kale, de-stemmed and chopped
- 1 tsp olive, coconut or canola oil
- Juice of 1/4 lime
- Garlic Roasted Broccoli:
- 2 cups broccoli,
- 2 tsp olive or canola oil
- 2 cloves garlic, minced
- Pinch of salt

- Black pepper
- Curry Roasted Sweet Potatoes:
- 1 small sweet potato
- 1 tsp olive or canola oil
- 1 tsp curry powder
- 1 tsp sriracha
- Pinch salt
- Spicy Roasted Chickpeas:
- 1 ½ cups (cooked) chickpeas
- 1 tsp olive or canola oil
- 2 tsp sriracha
- 2 tsp soy sauce
- Optional:
- Lime
- Avocado
- Hummus
- Red pepper flakes
- Guacamole

Directions:

- Preheat the oven to 400-degree F
- Line a large baking sheet with parchment paper
- Prepare the vegetables by chopping the broccoli into medium sized florets, de-stemming and chopping the kale, scrubbing and slicing the sweet potato into ¼" wide rounds
- Take the broccoli florets and massage with oil, garlic, salt and pepper - making sure to work the ingredients into the tops of each florets - Place the florets in a row down in the center third of a large baking sheet
- Using the same bowl, the broccoli in, mix together the chickpeas, oil, sriracha and soy sauce, then spread them out in a row next to the broccoli
- In the same bowl combine the oil, curry powder, salt, and sriracha, add the sliced sweet potato and toss to coat, then lay the rounds on the remaining third of the baking tray
- Bake for 10 minutes, flip the sweet potatoes and broccoli, and redistribute the chickpeas to cook evenly Bake for another 8-12 minutes
- For the Quinoa: Prepare the quinoa by rinsing and draining it. Add the rinsed quinoa and vegetable broth to a small saucepan and bring to a boil over high heat. Turn the heat down to medium-low, cover and allow to simmer for about 15 minutes. Once cooked, fluff with a fork and set aside
- In the meantime, place a large skillet with 1 tsp oil, add in the kale and cook for about 5 minutes, or until nearly tender
- Add in the salt, chili powder, and lime juice, toss to coat and cook for another 2-3 minutes
- Allow all the ingredient to cool
- Distribute among the containers – Add ½ to 1 cup of quinoa into each bowl, top with ½ of the broccoli, ½ kale, ½ the chickpeas and ½ sweet potatoes
- To Serve: Reheat in the microwave for 1-2 minutes or until heated through. Enjoy

Nutrition: Calories:611;Carbs: 93g;Total Fat: 17g;Protein: 24g

137) MEDITERRANEAN-STYLE SALMON

Cooking Time: 15 Minutes   **Servings: 4**

Ingredients:

- ½ cup of olive oil
- ¼ cup balsamic vinegar
- 4 garlic cloves, pressed
- 4 pieces salmon fillets

- 1 tbsp fresh cilantro, chopped
- 1 tbsp fresh basil, chopped
- 1½ tsp garlic salt

Directions:

- Combine olive oil and balsamic vinegar.
- Add salmon fillets to a shallow baking dish.
- Rub the garlic onto the fillets.
- Pour vinegar and oil all over, making sure to turn them once to coat them.
- Season with cilantro, garlic salt, and basil.
- Set aside and allow to marinate for about 10 minutes.
- Preheat the broiler to your oven.
- Place the baking dish with the salmon about 6 inches from the heat source.
- Broil for 15 minutes until both sides are evenly browned and can be flaked with a fork.
- Make sure to keep brushing with sauce from the pan.
- Enjoy!

Nutrition: Calories: 459, Total Fat: 36.2 g, Saturated Fat: 5.2 g, Cholesterol: 78 mg, Sodium: 80 mg, Total Carbohydrate: 1.2 g, Dietary Fiber: 0.1 g, Total Sugars: 0.1 g, Protein: 34.8 g, Vitamin D: 0 mcg, Calcium: 71 mg, Iron: 1 mg, Potassium: 710 mg

138) HEARTTHROB MEDITERRANEAN-STYLE TILAPIA

Cooking Time: 15 Minutes   **Servings:** 4

Ingredients:

- ✓ 3 tbsp sun-dried tomatoes, packed in oil, drained and chopped
- ✓ 1 tbsp capers, drained
- ✓ 2 tilapia fillets
- ✓ 1 tbsp oil from sun-dried tomatoes
- ✓ 1 tbsp lemon juice
- ✓ 2 tbsp kalamata olives, chopped and pitted

Directions:

- ❖ Pre-heat your oven to 372-degree Fahrenheit
- ❖ Take a small sized bowl and add sun-dried tomatoes, olives, capers and stir well
- ❖ Keep the mixture on the side
- ❖ Take a baking sheet and transfer the tilapia fillets and arrange them side by side
- ❖ Drizzle olive oil all over them
- ❖ Drizzle lemon juice
- ❖ Bake in your oven for 10-15 minutes
- ❖ After 10 minutes, check the fish for a "Flaky" texture
- ❖ Once cooked properly, top the fish with tomato mix and serve!
- ❖ Meal Prep/Storage Options: Store in airtight containers in your fridge for 1-3 days.

Nutrition: Calories: 183;Fat: 8g;Carbohydrates: 18g;Protein:183g

139) GARLIC WITH CAJUN SHRIMP BOWL AND NOODLES

Cooking Time: 15 Minutes   **Servings:** 2

Ingredients:

- ✓ 1 sliced onion
- ✓ 1 tbsp almond butter, but you can use regular butter as well
- ✓ 1 tsp onion powder
- ✓ ½ tsp salt
- ✓ 1 sliced red pepper
- ✓ 3 cloves of minced garlic
- ✓ 1 tsp paprika
- ✓ 20 jumbo shrimp, deveined and shells removed
- ✓ 3 tbsp of ghee
- ✓ 2 zucchini, 3 if they are smaller in size, cut into noodles
- ✓ Red pepper flakes and cayenne pepper, as desired

Directions:

- ❖ In a small bowl, mix the pepper flakes, paprika, onion powder, salt, and cayenne pepper.
- ❖ Toss the shrimp into the cajun mixture and coat the seafood thoroughly.
- ❖ Add the ghee to a medium or large skillet and place on medium-low heat.
- ❖ Once the ghee is melted, add the garlic and saute for minutes.
- ❖ Carefully add the shrimp into the skillet and cook until they are opaque. Set the pan aside.
- ❖ In a new pan, add the butter and allow it to melt.
- ❖ Combine the zucchini noodles and cook on medium-low heat for 3 to 4 minutes.
- ❖ Turn off the heat and place the zucchini noodles on serving dishes. Add the shrimp to the top and enjoy.

Nutrition: calories: 712, fats: 30 grams, carbohydrates: 20.1 grams, protein: grams.

140) MARINATED CHICKEN WITH GARLIC

Cooking Time: 15 Minutes   **Servings:** 3

Ingredients:

- ✓ 1 ½ lbs. boneless skinless chicken breasts,
- ✓ 1/4 cup olive oil
- ✓ 1/4 cup lemon juice
- ✓ 3 cloves garlic, minced
- ✓ 1/2 tbsp dried oregano
- ✓ 1/2 tsp salt
- ✓ Freshly cracked pepper
- ✓ To Serve:
- ✓ Rice or cauliflower rice
- ✓ Roasted vegetables, such as carrots, asparagus, or green beans

Directions:

- ❖ In a large Ziplock bag or dish, add in the olive oil, lemon juice, garlic, oregano, salt, and pepper
- ❖ Close the bag and shake the ingredients to combine, or stir the ingredients in the dish until well combined
- ❖ Filet each chicken breast into two thinner pieces and place the pieces in the bag or dish - make sure the chicken is completely covered in marinade and allow to marinate for up to minutes up to 8 hours, turn occasionally to maximize the marinade flavors
- ❖ Once ready, heat a large skillet over medium heat
- ❖ Once heated, transfer the chicken from the marinade to the hot skillet and cook on each side cooked through, about 7 minutes each side, depending on the size - Discard of any excess marinade
- ❖ Transfer the cooked chicken from the skillet to a clean cutting board, allow to rest for five minutes before slicing
- ❖ Distribute the chicken, cooked rice and vegetables among the containers. Store in the fridge for up to 4 days. To Serve: Reheat in the microwave for 1-2 minutes or until heated through and enjoy!

Nutrition: Calories:446;Total Fat: 24g;Total Carbs: 4g;Fiber: 0g;Protein: 52g

141) TABOULI SALAD

Cooking Time: 30 Minutes   **Servings:** 6

Ingredients:

- ½ cup extra fine bulgar wheat
- 4 firm Roma tomatoes, finely chopped, juice drained
- 1 English cucumber, finely chopped
- 2 bunches fresh parsley, stems removed, finely chopped
- 12-15 fresh mint leaves, finely chopped
- 4 green onions, finely chopped (white and green)
- salt
- 3-4 tbsp lime juice
- 3-4 tbsp extra virgin olive oil
- Romaine lettuce leaves
- pita bread

Directions:

- Wash bulgur wheat thoroughly and allow it to soak under water for 5 minutes.
- Drain bulgur wheat well and set aside.
- Add all vegetables, green onions, and herbs to a dish.
- Add bulgur and season the mixture with salt.
- Add limejuice and olive oil. Mix well.
- Put to the jars and refrigerate.
- Transfer to a serving platter and serve with sides of pita and romaine lettuce.

Nutrition: Calories: 136, Total Fat: 7.6 g, Saturated Fat: 1.1 g, Cholesterol: 0 mg, Sodium: 72 mg, Total Carbohydrate: 15.6 g, Dietary Fiber: 3.7 g, Total Sugars: 3.6 g, Protein: 3.4 g, Vitamin D: 0 mcg, Calcium: 71 mg, Iron: 3 mg, Potassium: 439 mg

142) MEDITERRANEAN-STYLE FLOUNDER

Cooking Time: 45 Minutes   **Servings:** 4

Ingredients:

- Roma or plum tomatoes (5)
- Extra-virgin olive oil (2 tbsp.)
- Spanish onion (half of 1)
- Garlic (2 cloves)
- Italian seasoning (1 pinch)
- Kalamata olives (24)
- White wine (.25 cup)
- Capers (.25 cup)
- Lemon juice (1 tsp.)
- Chopped basil (6 leaves)
- Freshly grated parmesan cheese (3 tbsp.)
- Flounder fillets (1 lb.)
- Freshly torn basil (6 leaves)

Directions:

- Set the oven to reach 425° Fahrenheit. Remove the pit and chop the olives (set aside.
- Pour water into a saucepan and bring to boiling. Plunge the tomatoes into the water and remove immediately. Add to a dish of ice water and drain. Remove the skins, chop, and set to the side for now.
- Heat a skillet with the oil using the medium temperature heat setting. Chop and toss in the onions. Sauté them for around four minutes.
- Dice and add the garlic, tomatoes, and seasoning. Simmer for five to seven minutes.
- Stir in the capers, wine, olives, half of the basil, and freshly squeezed lemon juice.
- Lower the heat setting and blend in the cheese. Simmer it until the sauce is thickened (15 min..
- Arrange the flounder into a shallow baking tin. Add the sauce and garnish with the remainder of the basil leaves.
- Set the timer to bake it for 12 minutes until the fish is easily flaked.

Nutrition: Calories: 282;Protein: 24.4 grams;Fat: 15.4 grams

143) LEMON GREEK CHICKEN SOUP

Cooking Time: 20 Minutes   **Servings:** 8

Ingredients:

- 10 cups chicken broth
- 3 tbsp olive oil
- 8 cloves garlic, minced
- 1 sweet onion
- 1 large lemon, zested
- 2 boneless skinless chicken breasts
- 1 cup Israeli couscous (pearl)
- 1/2 tsp crushed red pepper
- 2 oz crumbled feta
- 1/3 cup chopped chive
- Salt, to taste
- Pepper, to taste

Directions:

- In a large 6-8-quart sauce pot over medium-low heat, add the olive oil
- Once heated, sauté the onion and minced the garlic for 3-4 minutes to soften
- Then add in the chicken broth, raw chicken breasts, lemon zest, and crushed red pepper to the pot Raise the heat to high, cover, and bring to a boil
- Once boiling, reduce the heat to medium, then simmer for 5 minutes Stir in the couscous, 1 tsp salt, and black pepper to taste
- Simmer another 5 minute, then turn the heat off Using tongs, remove the two chicken breasts from the pot and transfer to a plate
- Use a fork and the tongs to shred the chicken, then return to the pot
- Stir in the crumbled feta cheese and chopped chive Season to taste with salt and pepper as needed
- Allow the soup to cool completely Distribute among the containers, store for 2-3 days
- To Serve: Reheat in the microwave for 1-2 minutes or until heated through, or reheat on the stove

Nutrition: Calories:2Carbs: 23g;Total Fat: g;Protein: 11g

144) MEDITERRANEAN-STYLE STEAMED SALMON WITH FRESH HERBS AND LEMON

Cooking Time: 15 Minutes   **Servings:** 4

Ingredients:

- ✓ 1 yellow onion, halved and sliced
- ✓ 4 green onions spring onions, trimmed and sliced lengthwise, divided
- ✓ 1 lb skin-on salmon fillet (such as wild Alaskan), cut into 4 portions
- ✓ 1/2 tsp Aleppo pepper
- ✓ 4 to 5 garlic cloves, chopped
- ✓ Extra virgin olive oil
- ✓ A large handful fresh parsley
- ✓ 1 lemon, thinly sliced
- ✓ 1 tsp ground coriander
- ✓ 1 tsp ground cumin
- ✓ 1/2 cup white wine (or you can use water or low-sodium broth, if you prefer)
- ✓ Kosher salt, to taste
- ✓ Black pepper, to taste

Directions:

- ❖ Prepare a large piece of wax paper or parchment paper (about 2 feet long) and place it right in the center of a -inch deep pan or braiser
- ❖ Place the sliced yellow onions and a sprinkle a little bit of green onions the onions on the bottom of the braiser
- ❖ Arrange the salmon, skin-side down, on top, season with kosher salt and black pepper
- ❖ In a small bowl, mix together the coriander, cumin, and Aleppo pepper, coat top of salmon with the spice mixture, and drizzle with a little bit of extra virgin olive oil
- ❖ Then add garlic, parsley and the remaining green onions on top of the salmon (make sure that everything is arrange evenly over the salmon portions.)
- ❖ Arrange the lemon slices on top of the salmon
- ❖ Add another drizzle of extra virgin olive oil, then add the white wine
- ❖ Fold the parchment paper over to cover salmon, secure the edges and cover the braiser with the lid
- ❖ Place the braising pan over medium-high heat, cook for 5 minutes
- ❖ Lower the heat to medium, cook for another 8 minutes, covered still
- ❖ Remove from heat and allow to rest undisturbed for about 5 minutes.
- ❖ Remove the lid and allow the salmon to cool completely
- ❖ Distribute among the containers, store for 2-3 days
- ❖ To Serve: Reheat in the microwave for 1-2 minutes or until heated through.
- ❖ Recipe Notes: The pan or braiser you use needs to have a lid to allow the steamed salmon.

Nutrition: Calories:321;Carbs: g;Total Fat: 18g;Protein: 28g

145) BEEF-BASED SAUSAGE PANCAKES

Cooking Time: 30 Minutes   **Servings:** 2

Ingredients:

- ✓ 4 gluten-free Italian beef sausages, sliced
- ✓ 1 tbsp olive oil
- ✓ 1/3 large red bell peppers, seeded and sliced thinly
- ✓ 1/3 cup spinach
- ✓ ¾ tsp garlic powder
- ✓ 1/3 large green bell peppers, seeded and sliced thinly
- ✓ ¾ cup heavy whipped cream
- ✓ Salt and black pepper, to taste

Directions:

- ❖ Mix together all the ingredients in a bowl except whipped cream and keep aside.
- ❖ Put butter and half of the mixture in a skillet and cook for about 6 minutes on both sides.
- ❖ Repeat with the remaining mixture and dish out.
- ❖ Beat whipped cream in another bowl until smooth.
- ❖ Serve the beef sausage pancakes with whipped cream.
- ❖ For meal prepping, it is compulsory to gently slice the sausages before mixing with other ingredients.

Nutrition: Calories: 415 ;Carbohydrates: ;Protein: 29.5g;Fat: 31.6g ;Sugar: 4.3g;Sodium: 1040mg

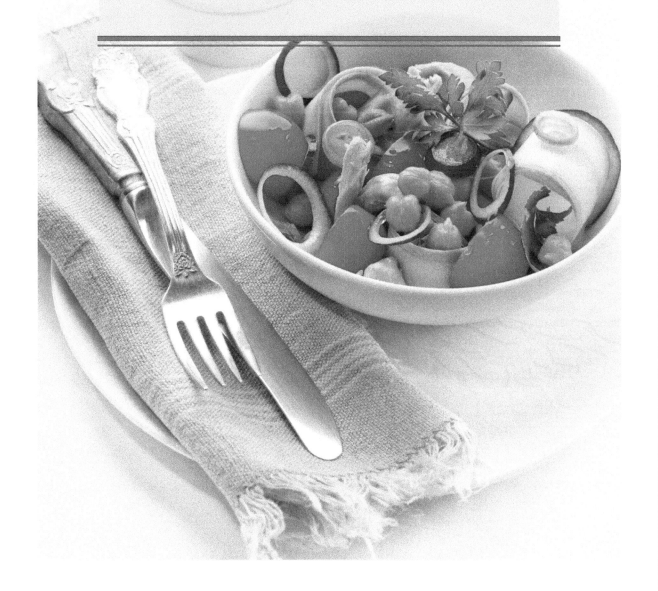

SOUPS & SALADS

146) TYPICAL BEEF STROGANOFF SOUP

Cooking Time: 35 Minutes   **Servings: 6**

Ingredients:

- 1.5 pounds stew meat
- 6 cups beef broth
- 4 tbsp Worcestershire sauce
- 1/2 tsp Italian seasoning blend
- 1 1/2 tsp onion powder
- 2 tsp garlic powder
- salt and pepper to taste
- 1/2 cup sour cream
- 8 ounces mushrooms, sliced
- 8 ounces short noodles, cooked
- 1/3 cup cold water
- 1/4 cup corn starch

Directions:

- Add meat, 5 cups broth, Italian seasoning, Worcestershire sauce, garlic powder, salt, pepper, and onion powder to the insert of the Instant Pot.
- Secure and seal the Instant Pot lid then select Manual mode for 1 hour at high pressure.
- Once done, release the pressure completely then remove the lid.
- Set the Instant pot on Soup mode and add sour cream along with 1 cup broth.
- Mix well then add mushrooms and mix well.
- Whisk corn-starch with water and pour this mixture into the pot.
- Cook this mixture until it thickens then add noodles, salt, and pepper.
- Garnish with cheese parsley, black pepper.
- Enjoy.

Nutrition: Calories: 320;Carbohydrate: 21.6g;Protein: 26.9g;Fat: 13.7g;Sugar: 7.1g;Sodium: 285mg

147) EGG, AVOCADO WITH TOMATO SALAD

Cooking Time: 40 Minutes   **Servings: 4**

Ingredients:

- 2 boiled eggs, chopped into chunks
- 1 ripe avocado, chopped into chunks
- 1 medium-sized tomato, chopped into chunks
- Salt and black pepper, to taste
- 1 lemon wedge, juiced

Directions:

- Mix together all the ingredients in a large bowl until well combined.
- Dish out in a glass bowl and serve immediately.

Nutrition: Calories: 140;Carbs: 5.9g;Fats: 12.1g;Proteins: 4g;Sodium: mg;Sugar: 1.3g

148) SPECIAL CREAMY LOW CARB BUTTERNUT SQUASH SOUP

Cooking Time: 1 Hour 10 Minutes   **Servings: 8**

Ingredients:

- 2 tbsp avocado oil, divided
- 2 pounds butternut squash, cut in half length-wise and seeds removed
- Sea salt and black pepper, to taste
- 1 (13.5-oz can coconut milk
- 4 cups chicken bone broth

Directions:

- Preheat the oven to 400 degrees F and grease a baking sheet.
- Arrange the butternut squash halves with open side up on the baking sheet.
- Drizzle with half of the avocado oil and season with sea salt and black pepper.
- Flip over and transfer into the oven.
- Roast the butternut squash for about minutes.
- Heat the remaining avocado oil over medium heat in a large pot and add the broth and coconut milk.
- Let it simmer for about 20 minutes and scoop the squash out of the shells to transfer into the soup.
- Puree this mixture in an immersion blender until smooth and serve immediately.

Nutrition: Calories: 185;Carbs: 12.6g;Fats: 12.6g;Proteins: 4.7g;Sodium: 3mg;Sugar: 4.5g

149) SPECIAL BUTTERNUT SQUASH SOUP

Cooking Time: 40 Minutes   **Servings:** 4

Ingredients:

- ✓ 1 tbsp olive oil
- ✓ 1 medium yellow onion chopped
- ✓ 1 large carrot chopped
- ✓ 1 celery rib chopped
- ✓ 3 cloves of garlic minced
- ✓ 2 lbs. butternut squash, peeled chopped
- ✓ 2 cups vegetable broth
- ✓ 1 green apple peeled, cored, and chopped
- ✓ 1/4 tsp ground cinnamon
- ✓ 1 sprig fresh thyme
- ✓ 1 sprig fresh rosemary
- ✓ 1 tsp kosher salt
- ✓ 1/2 tsp black pepper
- ✓ Pinch of nutmeg optional

Directions:

- ❖ Preheat olive oil in the insert of the Instant Pot on Sauté mode.
- ❖ Add celery, carrots, and garlic, sauté for 5 minutes.
- ❖ Stir in squash, broth, cinnamon, apple nutmeg, rosemary, thyme, salt, and pepper.
- ❖ Mix well gently then seal and secure the lid.
- ❖ Select Manual mode to cook for 10 minutes at high pressure.
- ❖ Once done, release the pressure completely then remove the lid.
- ❖ Puree the soup using an immersion blender.
- ❖ Serve warm.

Nutrition: Calories: 282;Carbohydrate: 50g;Protein: 13g;Fat: 4.7g;Sugar: 12.8g;Sodium: 213mg

150) LOVELY CREAMY CILANTRO LIME COLESLAW

Cooking Time: 10 Minutes   **Servings:** 2

Ingredients:

- ✓ ¾ avocado
- ✓ 1 lime, juiced
- ✓ 1/8 cup water
- ✓ Cilantro, to garnish
- ✓ 6 oz coleslaw, bagged
- ✓ 1/8 cup cilantro leaves
- ✓ 1 garlic clove
- ✓ ¼ tsp salt

Directions:

- ❖ Put garlic and cilantro in a food processor and process until chopped.
- ❖ Add lime juice, avocado and water and pulse until creamy.
- ❖ Put coleslaw in a large bowl and stir in the avocado mixture.
- ❖ Refrigerate for a few hours before serving.

Nutrition: Calories: 240;Carbs: 17.4g;Fats: 19.6g;Proteins: 2.8g;Sodium: 0mg;Sugar: 0.5g

151) CLASSIC SNAP PEA SALAD

Cooking Time: 15 Minutes   **Servings:** 2

Ingredients:

- ✓ 1/8 cup lemon juice
- ✓ ½ clove garlic, crushed
- ✓ 4 ounces cauliflower riced
- ✓ 1/8 cup olive oil
- ✓ ¼ tsp coarse grain Dijon mustard
- ✓ ½ tsp granulated stevia
- ✓ ¼ cup sugar snap peas, ends removed and each pod cut into three pieces
- ✓ 1/8 cup chives
- ✓ 1/8 cup red onions, minced
- ✓ Sea salt and black pepper, to taste
- ✓ ¼ cup almonds, sliced

Directions:

- ❖ Pour water in a pot fitted with a steamer basket and bring water to a boil.
- ❖ Place riced cauliflower in the steamer basket and season with sea salt.
- ❖ Cover the pot and steam for about 10 minutes until tender.
- ❖ Drain the cauliflower and dish out in a bowl to refrigerate for about 1 hour.
- ❖ Meanwhile, make a dressing by mixing olive oil, lemon juice, garlic, mustard, stevia, salt and black pepper in a bowl.
- ❖ Mix together chilled cauliflower, peas, chives, almonds and red onions in another bowl.
- ❖ Pour the dressing over this mixture and serve.

Nutrition: Calories: 203;Carbs: 7.6g;Fats: 18g;Proteins: 4.2g;Sodium: 28mg;Sugar: 2.9g

152) SPINACH AND BACON SALAD

Cooking Time: 15 Minutes   **Servings:** 4

Ingredients:

- ✓ 2 eggs, boiled, halved, and sliced
- ✓ 10 oz. organic baby spinach, rinsed, and dried
- ✓ 8 pieces thick bacon, cooked and sliced
- ✓ ½ cup plain mayonnaise
- ✓ ½ medium red onion, thinly sliced

Directions:

- ❖ Mix together the mayonnaise and spinach in a large bowl.
- ❖ Stir in the rest of the ingredients and combine well.
- ❖ Dish out in a glass bowl and serve well.

Nutrition: Calories: 373;Carbs: ;Fats: 34.5g;Proteins: 11g;Sodium: 707mg;Sugar: 1.1g

Sauces and Dressings Recipes

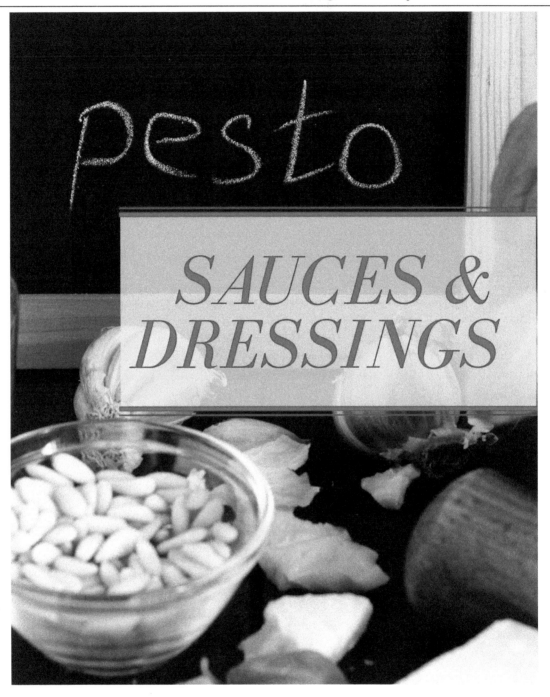

153) GREEK-STYLE SALAD

Preparation Time: 20 minutes   **Cooking Time:** 0 minute   **Servings: 5**

Ingredients:

- ✓ Dressing
- ✓ 6 tbsp olive oil
- ✓ ¾ tsp honey
- ✓ 1 tbsp red wine vinegar
- ✓ 1/5 tbsp lemon juice
- ✓ 1.5 tsp minced garlic
- ✓ 1 tsp oregano
- ✓ 1.5 tbsp minced parsley
- ✓ Salt to taste

- ✓ Salad
- ✓ Four diced tomatoes
- ✓ ½ chopped onion
- ✓ One chopped English cucumber
- ✓ One chopped green bell pepper
- ✓ 4 oz feta cheese
- ✓ ¾ cup sliced Kalamata olives
- ✓ One chopped avocado

Directions:

- ❖ Whisk all the ingredients mentioned in the dressing list in a large mixing bowl. Set aside.
- ❖ In another bowl, add all the ingredients of the salad and toss well.
- ❖ Pour the dressing, toss well and serve.

Nutrition: Calories: 248 kcal Fat: 24 g Protein: 3 g Carbs: 4 g Fiber: 1 g

154) LOVELY CREAMIEST HUMMUS

Preparation Time: 5 minutes   **Cooking Time:** 0 minute   **Servings: 10**

Ingredients:

- ✓ 400 g chickpeas
- ✓ ½ tsp salt
- ✓ 8 tbsp tahini

- ✓ 10 tbsp liquid from chickpeas can
- ✓ 2 tbsp lemon juice
- ✓ 1 tbsp olive oil

Directions:

- ❖ In a food processor, blend chickpeas, lemon juice, tahini, salt, and aquafaba to get smooth hummus.
- ❖ Transfer the blended hummus to the bowl. Pour olive oil in the center of the hummus and serve.

Nutrition: Calories: 100 kcal Fat: 7 g Protein: 3 g Carbs: 5 g Fiber: 3 g

155) ITALIAN ROASTED VEGETABLES

Preparation Time: 10 minutes   **Cooking Time:** 30 minutes   **Servings: 6**

Ingredients:

- ✓ 8 oz mushrooms
- ✓ 12 oz Campari tomatoes
- ✓ Extra virgin olive as required
- ✓ Two sliced zucchinis
- ✓ 12 oz sliced baby potatoes

- ✓ 11 chopped garlic cloves
- ✓ 1 tsp dried thyme
- ✓ Salt to taste
- ✓ Shredded Parmesan cheese
- ✓ Black pepper to taste
- ✓ ½ tbsp dried oregano
- ✓ Red pepper flakes to taste

Directions:

- ❖ Add salt, mushrooms, olive oil, pepper, veggies, oregano, garlic, and thyme in a mixing bowl and toss well. Set aside.
- ❖ Roast potatoes in a preheated oven at 425 degrees for 10 minutes.
- ❖ Mix the mushroom mixture with baked potatoes and bake for another 20 minutes.
- ❖ Garnish with cheese and pepper flakes and serve.

Nutrition: Calories: 88 kcal Fat: 1 g Protein: 3.8 g Carbs: 14.3 g Fiber: 3.1 g

156) SIMPLE WHITE BEAN SALAD

Preparation Time: 15 minutes   **Cooking Time:** 0 minute   **Servings: 4**

Ingredients:

- ✓ 2o oz white beans
- ✓ 10 oz halved cherry tomatoes
- ✓ One chopped English cucumber
- ✓ Four chopped onion
- ✓ 18 chopped mint leaves
- ✓ 1 cup chopped parsley

- ✓ 1 tbsp of lemon juice
- ✓ Salt to taste
- ✓ Zested of one lemon
- ✓ Black pepper to taste
- ✓ ½ tsp Sumac
- ✓ Feta cheese
- ✓ 1 tsp Za'atar
- ✓ ½ tsp Aleppo
- ✓ Olive oil

Directions:

- ❖ Combine all the ingredients in a large salad bowl and toss well to mix everything evenly.
- ❖ Serve and enjoy it.

Nutrition: Calories: 310 kcal Fat: 7 g Protein: 16 g Carbs: 47 g Fiber: 11 g

157) EASY ROASTED CAULIFLOWER WITH LEMON AND CUMIN

Preparation Time: 15 minutes   **Cooking Time:** 25 minutes   **Servings: 4**

Ingredients:

- 11 oz cauliflower
- 1 tbsp of lemon juice
- 1/3 cup olive oil
- Salt to taste
- Zest of one lemon
- 1 tbsp ground sumac
- 1 tbsp ground cumin
- 1 tsp garlic powder
- Black pepper to taste

Directions:

- Mix all the ingredients in a large mixing bowl.
- Transfer the cauliflower to a baking tray and bake in a preheated oven at 425 degrees for 25 minutes.
- Serve and enjoy it.

Nutrition: Calories: 213 kcal Fat: 18 g Protein: 3 g Carbs: 10 g Fiber: 3 g

158) SPECIAL TABBOULEH SALAD

Preparation Time: 20 minutes   **Cooking Time:** 0 minute   **Servings: 6**

Ingredients:

- ½ cup bulgur wheat
- One chopped English cucumber
- Four chopped tomatoes
- Two chopped parsley
- Four chopped green onions
- 13 chopped mint leaves
- Salt to taste
- 4 tbsp extra virgin olive oil
- 4 tbsp lime juice
- Romaine lettuce leaves to garnishing

Directions:

- Soak bulgur for 10 minutes in water.
- Drain to remove all the excess water and keep it aside.
- Now, mix all the ingredients in a large salad bowl and place them for 30 minutes in the refrigerator to get the best results.

Nutrition: Calories: 190 kcal Fat: 10 g Protein: 3.2 g Carbs: 25.5 g Fiber: 3.1 g

159) TASTY WATERMELON SALAD

Preparation Time: 15 minutes   **Cooking Time:** 0 minute   **Servings: 6**

Ingredients:

- Honey Vinaigrette
- 2 tbsp extra virgin olive oil
- 2 tbsp honey
- One pinch of salt
- ½ chopped watermelon
- Watermelon Salad
- 2 tbsp lime juice
- One chopped English cucumber
- 15 chopped basil leaves
- 15 chopped mint leaves
- ½ cup feta cheese

Directions:

- In a bowl, combine watermelon, herbs, and cucumber and set aside.
- In another bowl, mix oil, salt, honey, and lemon juice and pour the dressing into a watermelon bowl.
- Toss well and serve.

Nutrition: Calories: 192 kcal Fat: 5.6 g Protein: 4.3 g Carbs: 35.9 g Fiber: 11 g

160) SPECIAL LOADED CHICKPEA SALAD

Preparation Time: 20 minutes   **Cooking Time:** 10 minutes   **Servings: 6**

Ingredients:

- Olive oil
- One sliced eggplant
- 1 cup cooked chickpeas
- Three diced Roma tomatoes
- 3 tbsp Za'atar spice
- Salt to taste
- ½ chopped English cucumber
- 1 cup chopped parsley
- One chopped small red onion
- 1 cup chopped dill
- Garlic Vinaigrette
- Two chopped garlic cloves
- 1/3 cup extra virgin olive oil
- 2 tbsp lime juice
- Salt to taste
- Black pepper to taste

Directions:

- Season eggplant with salt and set aside for 30 minutes.
- Dry eggplant and cook in olive oil for five minutes from each side.
- When the eggplant has turned brown from both sides, remove the pan from the flame and keep it aside.
- In a bowl, combine cucumber, onions, tomatoes, dill, zaatar, chickpeas, parsley, and mix well.
- Place all the dressing ingredients in a bowl and toss well.
- Transfer cooked eggplant and chickpeas mixture in one large bowl and poured the dressing over them.
- Serve and enjoy it.

Nutrition: Calories: 308 kcal Fat: 15.3 g Protein: 11.1 g Carbs: 17.3 g Fiber: 9.6 g

161) ITALIAN BAKED ZUCCHINI WITH THYME AND PARMESAN

Preparation Time: 10 minutes   **Cooking Time:** 20 minutes   **Servings: 4**

Ingredients:

- Four sliced zucchinis
- 1/2 tsp dried thyme
- 1/2 cup shredded Parmesan cheese
- 1/2 tsp dried oregano
- 2 tbsp olive oil
- 1/4 tsp garlic powder
- Kosher salt to taste
- 1/2 tsp dried basil
- Black pepper to taste
- 2 tbsp chopped parsley

Directions:

- Mix all the ingredients in a large bowl except zucchini.
- Make a layer of zucchini over a baking sheet sprayed with oil.
- Transfer the cheese mixture over zucchini and pour olive oil over them.
- Bake in a preheated oven at 350 degrees for 15 minutes, followed by broiling for three minutes.
- Serve and enjoy it.

Nutrition: Calories: 151.3 kcal Fat: 11.2 g Protein: 7.4 g Carbs: 6.8 g Fiber: 2 g

162) MEDITERRANEAN BABA GANOUSH

Preparation Time: 10 minutes   **Cooking Time:** 40 minutes   **Servings: 4**

Ingredients:

- One eggplant
- 1 tbsp Greek yogurt
- olive oil
- 1.5 tbsp tahini paste
- 1 tbsp lime juice
- One garlic clove
- Salt to taste
- 1 tsp cayenne pepper
- Pepper to taste
- ½ tsp sumac for garnishing
- Parsley leaves for garnishing
- Toasted pine nuts for garnishing

Directions:

- Make slits in eggplant's skin.
- Place eggplant skin side upwards in a baking tray.
- Spray olive oil over eggplant.
- Bake in a preheated oven at 425 degrees for 40 minutes.
- Scoop the inner flesh of eggplant out and shift in a food processor. Add garlic, cayenne, yogurt, lime juice, salt, tahini, sumac, pepper, and blend. The baba ganoush is ready.
- You can refrigerator for better results for 60 minutes and sprinkle oil, sumac, parsley, and nuts and serve.

Nutrition: Calories: 114 kcal Fat: 7.7 g Protein: 2.8 g Carbs: 11.1 g Fiber: 5 g

163) SICILIAN SALMON FISH STICKS

Preparation Time: 10 minutes   **Cooking Time:** 18 minutes   **Servings: 4**

Ingredients:

- Fish Sticks
- 2 lb salmon fillet
- 1/4 tsp salt
- 1/4 tsp black pepper
- First coating
- 1/2 tsp garlic powder
- 1/2 tsp dried thyme
- 1 cup almond meal
- 1/2 tsp sea salt
- 1/4 tsp black pepper
- Second coating
- 1/2 tsp salt
- 2/3 cup chickpea flour
- Third coating
- Two eggs
- Dipping Sauce
- 1/4 tsp salt
- 1/4 cup Greek yogurt
- 1 tsp lemon juice
- 1 tbsp Dijon mustard
- 1/2 tsp dill
- 1/8 tsp garlic powder

Directions:

- Whisk all the ingredients for the dipping sauce list in a bowl and set aside. The dipping sauce is ready.
- Mix garlic, thyme, and almond meal in a bowl. The first coating is ready.
- Add chickpea flour in another bowl. The second coating is ready.
- Beat the eggs in another bowl. Set aside.
- Sprinkle pepper and salt over sliced fish with removed skin.
- First, coat the fish with chickpea flour, followed by coating with egg and almond meal coating.
- Aline coated fish pieces in a baking sheet covered with parchment paper.
- Bake in a preheated oven at 400 degrees for 18 minutes.
- Serve baked fish with dipping sauce and serve.

Nutrition: Calories: 92 kcal Fat: 5.7 g Protein: 14.4 g Carbs: 4.5 g Fiber: 1.3 g

164) AFRICAN BAKED FALAFEL

Preparation Time: 10 minutes   **Cooking Time:** 24 minutes   **Servings: 15 patties**

Ingredients:

- 15 oz chickpeas
- Three cloves garlic
- 1/4 cup chopped onion
- 1/2 cup parsley
- 2 tsp lemon juice
- 1/2 tsp baking soda
- 1 tbsp olive oil
- 1 tsp ground cumin
- 3/4 tsp salt
- 1 tsp coriander
- One pinch of cayenne
- 3 tbsp oat flour

Directions:

- Blend all the ingredients except oat flour and baking soda in a food processor to get roughly a blended mixture.
- Transfer the mixture to a bowl and add oat flour and baking soda. Using hands, mix the dough well.
- Make patties out of the falafel mixture and set aside for 15 minutes.
- Bake the falafel patties in a preheated oven at 375 degrees for 12 minutes and serve.

Nutrition: Calories: 143 kcal Fat: 5 g Protein: 6 g Carbs: 24 g Fiber: 6 g

165) CHIA GREEK YOGURT PUDDING

Preparation Time: 10 minutes   **Cooking Time:** 0 minute   **Servings: 4**

Ingredients:

- ✓ 1/8 tsp salt
- ✓ 1/4 cup chia seeds
- ✓ 3/4 cup milk
- ✓ Sliced almonds for garnishing
- ✓ 11 oz f Vanilla Yogurt
- ✓ 2 tbsp pure maple syrup
- ✓ 1 tsp vanilla extract

Directions:

- ❖ Whisk all the ingredients in a large bowl. Set aside for 24 hours in the refrigerator.
- ❖ Mix the mixture gently after 24 hours and serve after garnishing.

Nutrition: Calories: 179 kcal Fat: 5.6 g Protein: 10.1 g Carbs: 22.3 g Fiber: 6 g

166) MEDITERRANEAN-STYLE FARFALLE

Preparation Time: 10 minutes   **Cooking Time:** 15 minutes   **Servings: 7**

Ingredients:

- ✓ ½ cup pine nuts
- ✓ ½ cup shredded parmesan cheese
- ✓ 12 oz farfalle pasta
- ✓ Two chopped garlic cloves
- ✓ ½ cup olive oil
- ✓ 1 cup diced tomato
- ✓ ¼ cup chopped basil leaves
- ✓ ¼ cup red wine vinegar
- ✓ 1 lb crumbled chorizo sausage

Directions:

- ❖ In a saucepan, boil water with added salt.
- ❖ Add pasta and cook until pasta is done.
- ❖ In a pan, cook chorizo over medium flame. Stir in nuts and cook for five minutes.
- ❖ Mix garlic and cook for a minute before removing the pan from the flame.
- ❖ Transfer cooked pasta, vinegar, cheese, cooked chorizo mixture, olive oil, tomatoes, and basil. Mix well to coat everything and serve.

Nutrition: Calories: 692 kcal Fat: 48 g Protein: 26.9 g Carbs: 39.7 g Fiber: 15 g

167) POTATO WEDGES

Preparation Time: 5 minutes   **Cooking Time:** 30 minutes   **Servings: 4**

Ingredients:

- ✓ 1.5 tbsp olive oil
- ✓ ½ tsp chili powder
- ✓ Two wedges cut potatoes
- ✓ 1/8 black pepper
- ✓ ½ tsp salt
- ✓ ½ tsp paprika

Directions:

- ❖ Combine all the ingredients in a bowl.
- ❖ Transfer the mixture to an air fryer basket and cook in a preheated air fryer at 400 degrees for eight minutes from both sides.
- ❖ Serve and enjoy it.

Nutrition: Calories: 129 kcal Fat: g Protein: 2.3 g Carbs: 19 g Fiber: 11 g

168) ORIGINAL GREEK-STYLE POTATOES

Preparation Time: 20 minutes   **Cooking Time:** 120 minutes   **Servings: 4**

Ingredients:

- ✓ ¼ cup lemon juice
- ✓ 1 tsp rosemary
- ✓ 1/3 cup olive oil
- ✓ 1 tsp thyme
- ✓ Two chopped garlic cloves
- ✓ Two chicken bouillon cubes
- ✓ 1.5 cups water
- ✓ Six chopped potatoes
- ✓ Black pepper to taste

Directions:

- ❖ Mix all the ingredients in a large bowl and pour over the potatoes placed in the baking tray.
- ❖ Bake in a preheated oven at 350 degrees for 90 minutes.
- ❖ Serve and enjoy it.

Nutrition: Calories: 418 kcal Fat: 18.5 g Protein: 7 g Carbs: 58.6 g Fiber: 9 g

169) ITALIAN-STYLE CHICKEN WRAP

Preparation Time: 10 minutes   **Cooking Time:** 20 minutes   **Servings: 4**

Ingredients:

- ✓ Four flour tortillas
- ✓ Two sliced Roma tomatoes
- ✓ 2 tbsp butter
- ✓ 1/2 cup crushed croutons
- ✓ 1/2 cup mayonnaise
- ✓ 16 basil leaves
- ✓ 1/2 lb boneless chicken breasts
- ✓ 1/4 cup shredded Parmesan cheese
- ✓ 2 cups shredded romaine lettuce

Directions:

- ❖ Cook chicken over medium flame in melted butter for 20 minutes.
- ❖ Slice the chicken into strips.
- ❖ Whisk cheese and mayonnaise and pour over the tortilla.
- ❖ Place lettuce followed by chicken, basil, tomato, and croutons on tortilla and wrap.
- ❖ Serve and enjoy it.

Nutrition: Calories: 610 kcal Fat: 36 g Protein: 27 g Carbs: 42 g Fiber: 3 g

170) EASY SKINNY SLOW COOKER KALE AND TURKEY MEATBALL SOUP

Preparation Time: 15 minutes   **Cooking Time:** 240 minutes   **Servings: 4**

Ingredients:

- ¼ cup milk
- 1 lb lean turkey
- Two slices of bread
- One chopped shallot
- ½ tsp grated nutmeg
- Two chopped garlic cloves
- 1 tsp oregano
- Kosher salt to taste
- 1/4 tsp red pepper flakes
- Black pepper to taste
- 2 tbsp chopped parsley
- ½ cup grated Parmigiano-Reggiano
- One egg
- 8 cups chicken broth
- 1 tbsp olive oil
- 15 oz white beans
- ½ chopped onion
- Two sliced carrots
- 4 cups kale

Directions:

- Soak pieces of bread in milk in a bowl followed by the addition of nutmeg, flakes, cheese, turkey, parsley, shallot, oregano, salt, egg, garlic, and pepper.
- Mix well using hands. Make meatballs out of the turkey mixture.
- Fry meatballs in heat olive oil in a skillet over a high flame. Keep the fried meatballs aside for a few minutes.
- Place beans, onions, carrot, kale, and broth in a slow cooker, followed by adding meatballs in broth.
- Cover the cooker and cook for four hours.
- Garnish with grated cheese, parsley, and flakes and serve.

Nutrition: Calories: 297 kcal Fat: 10 g Protein: 21 g Carbs: 27 g Fiber: 2 g

171) SPECIAL CHICKEN CAPRESE SANDWICH

Preparation Time: 10 minutes   **Cooking Time:** 6 minutes   **Servings: 4**

Ingredients:

- 4 tbsp olive oil
- 1 tbsp lemon juice
- ¼ cup basil leaves
- 1 tsp minced parsley
- Kosher salt to taste
- Two boneless chicken breasts
- Black pepper to taste
- 10 oz sliced sourdough bread
- Eleven Campari tomatoes
- 8 oz sliced mozzarella cheese
- Balsamic vinegar as required

Directions:

- Add chicken pieces, olive oil, lemon juice, salt, parsley, and pepper in a bowl. Toss well to coat chicken evenly. Set aside.
- Grill the chicken on a preheated grill on a medium flame for six minutes from both sides.
- Toast the bread drizzled with olive oil.
- Sliced the bread into three pieces.
- Place chicken pieces, cheese, and tomato slices over each slice of bread.
- Sprinkle vinegar, oil, salt, basil, and pepper over the bread slices and serve.

Nutrition: Calories: 612.73 kcal Fat: 32.06 g Protein: 34.4 g Carbs: 46.88 g Fiber: 2.25 g

172) ORIGINAL MINESTRONE

Preparation Time: 15 minutes   **Cooking Time:** 30 minutes   **Servings: 6**

Ingredients:

- 2 tbsp olive oil
- 1/3 cup shredded parmesan cheese
- Four chopped garlic cloves
- One chopped onion
- Two chopped celery stalks
- 1/3 lb green beans
- One diced carrot
- 1 tsp oregano
- Salt to taste
- 1 tsp basil
- Black pepper to taste
- 14 oz crushed tomatoes
- 28 oz diced tomatoes
- 6 cups chicken stock
- 1 cup elbow pasta
- 15 oz beans
- 2 tbsp chopped basil

Directions:

- Sauté onions in heated olive oil over medium flame for five minutes.
- Stir in garlic and cook for half a minute.
- Mix carrot and celery and cook for five more minutes with occasional stirring.
- Add oregano, beans, salt, basil, and black pepper and cook for another three minutes with constant stirring.
- Pour broth followed by the addition of tomatoes and let it boil.
- Lower the flame to low and let it simmer for ten minutes.
- Add pasta and kidney beans and cook for another ten minutes. Mix salt and serve after garnishing with cheese and bail.

Nutrition: Calories: 260 kcal Fat: 8 g Protein: 15 g Carbs: 37 g Fiber: 10 g

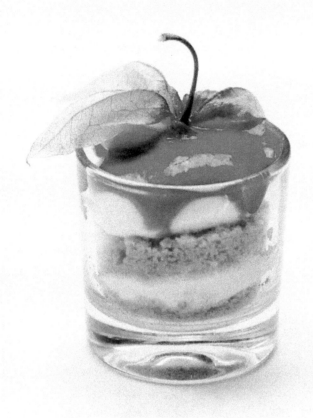

DESSERTS & SNACKS

173)   CLASSIC STUFFED FIGS

Cooking Time: 20 Minutes   **Servings: 6**

Ingredients:

- ✓ 10 halved fresh figs
- ✓ 20 chopped almonds
- ✓ 4 ounces goat cheese, divided
- ✓ 2 tbsp of raw honey

Directions:

- ❖ Turn your oven to broiler mode and set it to a high temperature.
- ❖ Place your figs, cut side up, on a baking sheet. If you like to place a piece of parchment paper on top you can do this, but it is not necessary.
- ❖ Sprinkle each fig with half of the goat cheese.
- ❖ Add a tbsp of chopped almonds to each fig.
- ❖ Broil the figs for 3 to 4 minutes.
- ❖ Take them out of the oven and let them cool for 5 to 7 minutes.
- ❖ Sprinkle with the remaining goat cheese and honey.

Nutrition: calories: 209, fats: 9 grams, carbohydrates: 26 grams, protein: grams.

174)   CHIA PUDDING AND STRAWBERRIES

Cooking Time: 4 Hours 5 Minutes   **Servings: 4**

Ingredients:

- ✓ 2 cups unsweetened almond milk
- ✓ 1 tbsp vanilla extract
- ✓ 2 tbsp raw honey
- ✓ ¼ cup chia seeds
- ✓ 2 cups fresh and sliced strawberries

Directions:

- ❖ In a medium bowl, combine the honey, chia seeds, vanilla, and unsweetened almond milk. Mix well.
- ❖ Set the mixture in the refrigerator for at least 4 hours.
- ❖ When you serve the pudding, top it with strawberries. You can even create a design in a glass serving bowl or dessert dish by adding a little pudding on the bottom, a few strawberries, top the strawberries with some more pudding, and then top the dish with a few strawberries.

Nutrition: calories: 108, fats: grams, carbohydrates: 17 grams, protein: 3 grams

175)   SPECIAL CHUNKY MONKEY TRAIL MIX

Cooking Time: 1 Hour 30 Minutes   **Servings: 6**

Ingredients:

- ✓ 1 cup cashews, halved
- ✓ 2 cups raw walnuts, chopped or halved
- ✓ ⅓ cup coconut sugar
- ✓ ½ cup of chocolate chips
- ✓ 1 tsp vanilla extract
- ✓ 1 cup coconut flakes, unsweetened and make sure you have big flakes and not shredded
- ✓ 6 ounces dried banana slices
- ✓ 1 ½ tsp coconut oil at room temperature

Directions:

- ❖ Turn your crockpot to high and add the cashews, walnuts, vanilla, coconut oil, and sugar. Combine until the ingredients are well mixed and then cook for 45 minutes.
- ❖ Reduce the temperature on your crockpot to low.
- ❖ Continue to cook the mixture for another 20 minutes.
- ❖ Place a piece of parchment paper on your counter.
- ❖ Once the mix is done cooking, remove it from the crockpot and set on top of the parchment paper.
- ❖ Let the mixture sit and cool for 20 minutes.
- ❖ Pour the contents into a bowl and add the dried bananas and chocolate chips. Gently mix the ingredients together. You can store the mixture in Ziplock bags for a quick and easy snack.

Nutrition: calories: 250, fats: 6 grams, carbohydrates: 1grams, protein: 4 grams

176) LOVELY STRAWBERRY POPSICLE

Cooking Time: 10 Minutes   **Servings: 5**

Ingredients:

✓ ½ cup almond milk

✓ 1 ½ cups fresh strawberries

Directions:

❖ Using a blender or hand mixer, combine the almond milk and strawberries thoroughly in a bowl.

❖ Using popsicle molds, pour the mixture into the molds and place the sticks into the mixture.

❖ Set in the freezer for at least 4 hours.

❖ Serve and enjoy—especially on a hot day!

Nutrition: calories: 3 fats: 0.5 grams, carbohydrates: 7 grams, protein: 0.6 grams.

177) SPECIAL FROZEN BLUEBERRY YOGURT

Cooking Time: 30 Minutes   **Servings: 6**

Ingredients:

✓ ⅔ cup honey
✓ 2 cups chilled yogurt
✓ 1 pint fresh blueberries

✓ 1 juiced and zested lime or lemon. You can even substitute an orange if your tastes prefer.

Directions:

❖ With a saucepan on your burner set to medium heat, add the honey, juiced fruit, zest, and blueberries.

❖ Stir the mixture continuously as it begins to simmer for 15 minutes.

❖ When the liquid is nearly gone, pour the contents into a bowl and place in the fridge for several minutes. You will want to stir the ingredients and check to see if they are chilled.

❖ Once the fruit is chilled, combine with the yogurt.

❖ Mix until the ingredients are well incorporated and enjoy.

Nutrition: calories: 233, fats: 3 grams, carbohydrates: 52 grams, protein: 3.5 grams

178) Delicious Almond Shortbread Cookies

Cooking Time: 25 Minutes   **Servings: 16**

Ingredients:

✓ ½ cup coconut oil
✓ 1 tsp vanilla extract
✓ 2 egg yolks
✓ 1 tbsp brandy
✓ 1 cup powdered sugar

✓ 1 cup finely ground almonds
✓ 3 ½ cups cake flour
✓ ½ cup almond butter
✓ 1 tbsp water or rose flower water

Directions:

❖ In a large bowl, combine the coconut oil, powdered sugar, and butter. If the butter is not soft, you want to wait until it softens up. Use an electric mixer to beat the ingredients together at high speed.

❖ In a small bowl, add the egg yolks, brandy, water, and vanilla extract. Whisk well.

❖ Fold the egg yolk mixture into the large bowl.

❖ Add the flour and almonds. Fold and mix with a wooden spoon.

❖ Place the mixture into the fridge for at least 1 hour and 30 minutes.

❖ Preheat your oven to 325 degrees Fahrenheit.

❖ Take the mixture, which now looks like dough, and divide it into 1-inch balls.

❖ With a piece of parchment paper on a baking sheet, arrange the cookies and flatten them with a fork or your fingers.

❖ Place the cookies in the oven for 13 minutes, but watch them so they don't burn.

❖ Transfer the cookies onto a rack to cool for a couple of minutes before enjoying!

Nutrition: calories: 250, fats: 14 grams, carbohydrates: 30 grams, protein: 3 grams

179)   CLASSIC CHOCOLATE FRUIT KEBABS

Cooking Time: 30 Minutes   **Servings: 6**

Ingredients:

- ✓ 24 blueberries
- ✓ 12 strawberries with the green leafy top part removed
- ✓ 12 green or red grapes, seedless
- ✓ 12 pitted cherries
- ✓ 8 ounces chocolate

Directions:

- ❖ Line a baking sheet with a piece of parchment paper and place 6, -inch long wooden skewers on top of the paper.
- ❖ Start by threading a piece of fruit onto the skewers. You can create and follow any pattern that you like with the ingredients. An example pattern is 1 strawberry, 1 cherry, blueberries, 2 grapes. Repeat the pattern until all of the fruit is on the skewers.
- ❖ In a saucepan on medium heat, melt the chocolate. Stir continuously until the chocolate has melted completely.
- ❖ Carefully scoop the chocolate into a plastic sandwich bag and twist the bag closed starting right above the chocolate.
- ❖ Snip the corner of the bag with scissors.
- ❖ Drizzle the chocolate onto the kebabs by squeezing it out of the bag.
- ❖ Put the baking pan into the freezer for 20 minutes.
- ❖ Serve and enjoy!

Nutrition: calories: 254, fats: 15 grams, carbohydrates: 28 grams, protein: 4 grams.

180)   CHERRY BROWNIES AND WALNUTS

Cooking Time: 25 To 30 Minutes   **Servings: 9**

Ingredients:

- ✓ 9 fresh cherries that are stemmed and pitted or 9 frozen cherries
- ✓ ½ cup sugar or sweetener substitute
- ✓ ¼ cup extra virgin olive oil
- ✓ 1 tsp vanilla extract
- ✓ ¼ tsp sea salt
- ✓ ½ cup whole-wheat pastry flour
- ✓ ¼ tsp baking powder
- ✓ ⅓ cup walnuts, chopped
- ✓ 2 eggs
- ✓ ½ cup plain Greek yogurt
- ✓ ⅓ cup cocoa powder, unsweetened

Directions:

- ❖ Make sure one of the metal racks in your oven is set in the middle.
- ❖ Turn the temperature on your oven to 375 degrees Fahrenheit.
- ❖ Using cooking spray, grease a 9-inch square pan.
- ❖ Take a large bowl and add the oil and sugar or sweetener substitute. Whisk the ingredients well.
- ❖ Add the eggs and use a mixer to beat the ingredients together.
- ❖ Pour in the yogurt and continue to beat the mixture until it is smooth.
- ❖ Take a medium bowl and combine the cocoa powder, flour, sea salt, and baking powder by whisking them together.
- ❖ Combine the powdered ingredients into the wet ingredients and use your electronic mixer to incorporate the ingredients together thoroughly.
- ❖ Add in the walnuts and stir.
- ❖ Pour the mixture into the pan.
- ❖ Sprinkle the cherries on top and push them into the batter. You can use any design, but it is best to make three rows and three columns with the cherries. This ensures that each piece of the brownie will have one cherry.
- ❖ Put the batter into the oven and turn your timer to 20 minutes.
- ❖ Check that the brownies are done using the toothpick test before removing them from the oven. Push the toothpick into the middle of the brownies and once it comes out clean, remove the brownies.
- ❖ Let the brownies cool for 5 to 10 minutes before cutting and serving.

181) SPECIAL FRUIT DIP

Cooking Time: 10 To 15 Minutes   **Servings: 10**

Ingredients:

- ✓ ¼ cup coconut milk, full-fat is best
- ✓ ¼ cup vanilla yogurt
- ✓ ⅓ cup marshmallow creme
- ✓ 1 cup cream cheese, set at room temperature
- ✓ 2 tbsp maraschino cherry juice

Directions:

- ❖ In a large bowl, add the coconut milk, vanilla yogurt, marshmallow creme, cream cheese, and cherry juice.
- ❖ Using an electric mixer, set to low speed and blend the ingredients together until the fruit dip is smooth.
- ❖ Serve the dip with some of your favorite fruits and enjoy!

Nutrition: calories: 110, fats: 11 grams, carbohydrates: 3 grams, protein: 3 grams

182) DELICIOUS LEMONY TREAT

Cooking Time: 30 Minutes   **Servings: 4**

Ingredients:

- ✓ 1 lemon, medium in size
- ✓ 1 ½ tsp cornstarch
- ✓ 1 cup Greek yogurt, plain is best
- ✓ Fresh fruit
- ✓ ¼ cup cold water
- ✓ ⅔ cup heavy whipped cream
- ✓ 3 tbsp honey
- ✓ Optional: mint leaves

Directions:

- ❖ Take a large glass bowl and your metal, electric mixer and set them in the refrigerator so they can chill.
- ❖ In a separate bowl, add the yogurt and set that in the fridge.
- ❖ Zest the lemon into a medium bowl that is microwavable.
- ❖ Cut the lemon in half and then squeeze 1 tbsp of lemon juice into the bowl.
- ❖ Combine the cornstarch and water. Mix the ingredients thoroughly.
- ❖ Pour in the honey and whisk the ingredients together.
- ❖ Put the mixture into the microwave for 1 minute on high.
- ❖ Once the microwave stops, remove the mixture and stir.
- ❖ Set it back into the microwave for 15 to 30 seconds or until the mixture starts to bubble and thicken.
- ❖ Take the bowl of yogurt from the fridge and pour in the warm mixture while whisking.
- ❖ Put the yogurt mixture back into the fridge.
- ❖ Take the large bowl and beaters out of the fridge.
- ❖ Put your electronic mixer together and pour the whipped cream into the chilled bowl.
- ❖ Beat the cream until soft peaks start to form. This can take up to 3 minutes, depending on how fresh your cream is.
- ❖ Remove the yogurt from the fridge.
- ❖ Fold the yogurt into the cream using a rubber spatula. Remember to lift and turn the mixture so it doesn't deflate.
- ❖ Place back into the fridge until you are serving the dessert or for 15 minutes. The dessert should not be in the fridge for longer than 1 hour.
- ❖ When you serve the lemony goodness, you will spoon it into four dessert dishes and drizzle with extra honey or even melt some chocolate to drizzle on top.
- ❖ Add a little fresh mint and enjoy!

Nutrition: calories: 241, fats: 16 grams, carbohydrates: 21 grams, protein: 7 grams

Meat Recipes

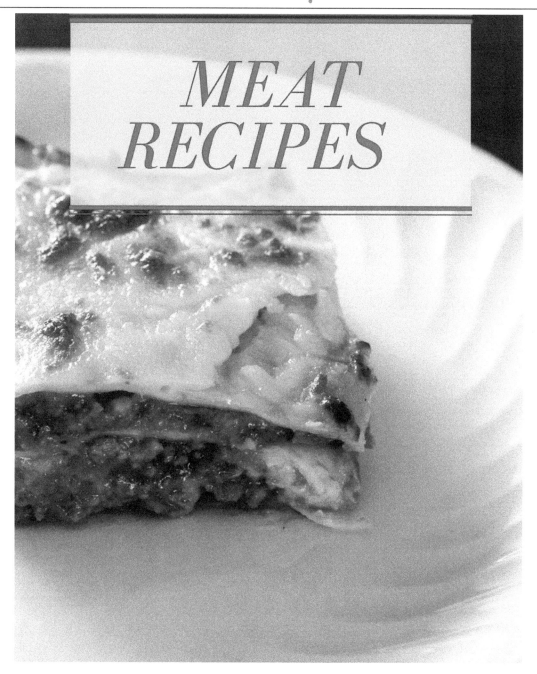

183) **CLASSIC TURKEY WINGS WITH GRAVY SAUCE**

Cooking Time: 6 Hours   **Servings: 6**

Ingredients:

- ✓ 2 pounds turkey wings
- ✓ 1/2 tsp cayenne pepper
- ✓ 4 garlic cloves, sliced
- ✓ 1 large onion, chopped
- ✓ Salt and pepper, to taste
- ✓ 1 tsp dried marjoram
- ✓ 1 tbsp butter, room temperature
- ✓ 1 tbsp Dijon mustard
- ✓ For the Gravy:
- ✓ 1 cup double cream
- ✓ Salt and black pepper, to taste
- ✓ 1/2 stick butter
- ✓ 3/4 tsp guar gum

Directions:

- ❖ Rub the turkey wings with the Dijon mustard and tbsp of butter. Preheat a grill pan over medium-high heat.
- ❖ Sear the turkey wings for 10 minutes on all sides.
- ❖ Transfer the turkey to your Crock pot; add in the garlic, onion, salt, pepper, marjoram, and cayenne pepper. Cover and cook on low setting for 6 hours.
- ❖ Melt 1/2 stick of the butter in a frying pan. Add in the cream and whisk until cooked through.
- ❖ Next, stir in the guar gum, salt, and black pepper along with cooking juices. Let it cook until the sauce has reduced by half.
- ❖ Storing
- ❖ Wrap the turkey wings in foil before packing them into airtight containers; keep in your refrigerator for up to 3 to 4 days.
- ❖ For freezing, place the turkey wings in airtight containers or heavy-duty freezer bags. Freeze up to 2 to 3 months. Defrost in the refrigerator.
- ❖ Keep your gravy in refrigerator for up to 2 days.

Nutrition: 280 Calories; 22.2g Fat; 4.3g Carbs; 15.8g Protein; 0.8g Fiber

184) AUTHENTIC PORK CHOPS WITH HERBS

Cooking Time: 20 Minutes   **Servings:** 4

Ingredients:

- ✓ 1 tbsp butter
- ✓ 1 pound pork chops
- ✓ 2 rosemary sprigs, minced
- ✓ 1 tsp dried marjoram
- ✓ 1 tsp dried parsley
- ✓ A bunch of spring onions, roughly chopped
- ✓ 1 thyme sprig, minced
- ✓ 1/2 tsp granulated garlic
- ✓ 1/2 tsp paprika, crushed
- ✓ Coarse salt and ground black pepper, to taste

Directions:

- ❖ Season the pork chops with the granulated garlic, paprika, salt, and black pepper.
- ❖ Melt the butter in a frying pan over a moderate flame. Cook the pork chops for 6 to 8 minutes, turning them occasionally to ensure even cooking.
- ❖ Add in the remaining ingredients and cook an additional 4 minutes.
- ❖ Storing
- ❖ Divide the pork chops into four portions; place each portion in a separate airtight container or Ziploc bag; keep in your refrigerator for 3 to 4 days.
- ❖ Freeze the pork chops in airtight containers or heavy-duty freezer bags. Freeze up to 4 months. Defrost in the refrigerator. Bon appétit!

Nutrition: 192 Calories; 6.9g Fat; 0.9g Carbs; 29.8g Protein; 0.4g Fiber

185) ORIGINAL GROUND PORK STUFFED PEPPERS

Cooking Time: 40 Minutes   **Servings:** 4

Ingredients:

- ✓ 6 bell peppers, deveined
- ✓ 1 tbsp vegetable oil
- ✓ 1 shallot, chopped
- ✓ 1 garlic clove, minced
- ✓ 1/2 pound ground pork
- ✓ 1/3 pound ground veal
- ✓ 1 ripe tomato, chopped
- ✓ 1/2 tsp mustard seeds
- ✓ Sea salt and ground black pepper, to taste

Directions:

- ❖ Parboil the peppers for 5 minutes.
- ❖ Heat the vegetable oil in a frying pan that is preheated over a moderate heat. Cook the shallot and garlic for 3 to 4 minutes until they've softened.
- ❖ Stir in the ground meat and cook, breaking apart with a fork, for about 6 minutes. Add the chopped tomatoes, mustard seeds, salt, and pepper.
- ❖ Continue to cook for 5 minutes or until heated through. Divide the filling between the peppers and transfer them to a baking pan.
- ❖ Bake in the preheated oven at 36degrees F approximately 25 minutes.
- ❖ Storing
- ❖ Place the peppers in airtight containers or Ziploc bags; keep in your refrigerator for up to 3 to 4 days.
- ❖ For freezing, place the peppers in airtight containers or heavy-duty freezer bags. Freeze up to 2 to 3 months. Defrost in the refrigerator. Bon appétit!

Nutrition: 2 Calories; 20.5g Fat; 8.2g Carbs; 18.2g Protein; 1.5g Fiber

186) GRILL-STYLE CHICKEN SALAD WITH AVOCADO

Cooking Time: 20 Minutes   **Servings: 4**

Ingredients:

- ✓ 1/3 cup olive oil
- ✓ 2 chicken breasts
- ✓ Sea salt and crushed red pepper flakes
- ✓ 2 egg yolks
- ✓ 1 tbsp fresh lemon juice
- ✓ 1/2 tsp celery seeds
- ✓ 1 tbsp coconut aminos
- ✓ 1 large-sized avocado, pitted and sliced

Directions:

- ❖ Grill the chicken breasts for about 4 minutes per side. Season with salt and pepper, to taste.
- ❖ Slice the grilled chicken into bite-sized strips.
- ❖ To make the dressing, whisk the egg yolks, lemon juice, celery seeds, olive oil and coconut aminos in a measuring cup.
- ❖ Storing
- ❖ Place the chicken breasts in airtight containers or Ziploc bags; keep in your refrigerator for 3 to 4 days.
- ❖ For freezing, place the chicken breasts in airtight containers or heavy-duty freezer bags. It will maintain the best quality for about 4 months. Defrost in the refrigerator.
- ❖ Store dressing in your refrigerator for 3 to 4 days. Dress the salad and garnish with fresh avocado. Bon appétit!

Nutrition: 40Calories; 34.2g Fat; 4.8g Carbs; 22.7g Protein; 3.1g Fiber

187) EASY-COOKING FALL-OFF-THE-BONE RIBS

Cooking Time: 8 Hours   **Servings: 4**

Ingredients:

- ✓ 1 pound baby back ribs
- ✓ 4 tbsp coconut aminos
- ✓ 1/4 cup dry red wine
- ✓ 1/2 tsp cayenne pepper
- ✓ 1 garlic clove, crushed
- ✓ 1 tsp Italian herb mix
- ✓ 1 tbsp butter
- ✓ 1 tsp Serrano pepper, minced
- ✓ 1 Italian pepper, thinly sliced
- ✓ 1 tsp grated lemon zest

Directions:

- ❖ Butter the sides and bottom of your Crock pot. Place the pork and peppers on the bottom.
- ❖ Add in the remaining ingredients.
- ❖ Slow cook for 9 hours on Low heat setting.
- ❖ Storing
- ❖ Divide the baby back ribs into four portions. Place each portion of the ribs along with the peppers in an airtight container; keep in your refrigerator for 3 to days.
- ❖ For freezing, place the ribs in airtight containers or heavy-duty freezer bags. Freeze up to 4 to months. Defrost in the refrigerator. Reheat in your oven at 250 degrees F until heated through.

Nutrition: 192 Calories; 6.9g Fat; 0.9g Carbs; 29.8g Protein; 0.5g Fiber

188) CLASSIC BRIE-STUFFED MEATBALLS

Cooking Time: 25 Minutes   **Servings: 5**

Ingredients:

- ✓ 2 eggs, beaten
- ✓ 1 pound ground pork
- ✓ 1/3 cup double cream
- ✓ 1 tbsp fresh parsley
- ✓ Kosher salt and ground black pepper
- ✓ 1 tsp dried rosemary
- ✓ 10 (1-inch cubes of brie cheese
- ✓ 2 tbsp scallions, minced
- ✓ 2 cloves garlic, minced

Directions:

- ❖ Mix all ingredients, except for the brie cheese, until everything is well incorporated.
- ❖ Roll the mixture into 10 patties; place a piece of cheese in the center of each patty and roll into a ball.
- ❖ Roast in the preheated oven at 0 degrees F for about 20 minutes.
- ❖ Storing
- ❖ Place the meatballs in airtight containers or Ziploc bags; keep in your refrigerator for up to 3 to 4 days.
- ❖ Freeze the meatballs in airtight containers or heavy-duty freezer bags. Freeze up to 3 to 4 months. To defrost, slowly reheat in a saucepan. Bon appétit!

Nutrition: 302 Calories; 13g Fat; 1.9g Carbs; 33.4g Protein; 0.3g Fiber

189) SPECIAL SPICY AND TANGY CHICKEN DRUMSTICKS

Cooking Time: 55 Minutes   **Servings: 6**

Ingredients:

- ✓ 3 chicken drumsticks, cut into chunks
- ✓ 1/2 stick butter
- ✓ 2 eggs
- ✓ 1/4 cup hemp seeds, ground
- ✓ Salt and cayenne pepper, to taste
- ✓ 2 tbsp coconut aminos
- ✓ 3 tsp red wine vinegar
- ✓ 2 tbsp salsa
- ✓ 2 cloves garlic, minced

Directions:

- ❖ Rub the chicken with the butter, salt, and cayenne pepper.
- ❖ Drizzle the chicken with the coconut aminos, vinegar, salsa, and garlic. Allow it to stand for 30 minutes in your refrigerator.
- ❖ Whisk the eggs with the hemp seeds. Dip each chicken strip in the egg mixture. Place the chicken chunks in a parchment-lined baking pan.
- ❖ Roast in the preheated oven at 390 degrees F for 25 minutes.
- ❖ Storing
- ❖ Divide the roasted chicken between airtight containers; keep in your refrigerator for up 3 to 4 days.
- ❖ For freezing, place the roasted chicken in airtight containers or heavy-duty freezer bags. Freeze up to 3 months. Defrost in the refrigerator and reheat in a pan. Enjoy!

Nutrition: 420 Calories; 22g Fat; 5g Carbs; 35.3g Protein; 0.8g Fiber

190) ORIGINAL ITALIAN-STYLE CHICKEN MEATBALLS WITH PARMESAN

Cooking Time: 20 Minutes   **Servings: 6**

Ingredients:

- ✓ For the Meatballs:
- ✓ 1 ¼ pounds chicken, ground
- ✓ 1 tbsp sage leaves, chopped
- ✓ 1 tsp shallot powder
- ✓ 1 tsp porcini powder
- ✓ 2 garlic cloves, finely minced
- ✓ 1/3 tsp dried basil
- ✓ 3/4 cup Parmesan cheese, grated
- ✓ 2 eggs, lightly beaten
- ✓ Salt and ground black pepper, to your liking
- ✓ 1/2 tsp cayenne pepper
- ✓ For the sauce:
- ✓ 2 tomatoes, pureed
- ✓ 1 cup chicken consommé
- ✓ 2 ½ tbsp lard, room temperature
- ✓ 1 onion, peeled and finely chopped

Directions:

- ❖ In a mixing bowl, combine all ingredients for the meatballs. Roll the mixture into bite-sized balls.
- ❖ Melt 1 tbsp of lard in a skillet over a moderately high heat. Sear the meatballs for about 3 minutes or until they are thoroughly cooked; reserve.
- ❖ Melt the remaining lard and cook the onions until tender and translucent. Add in pureed tomatoes and chicken consommé and continue to cook for 4 minutes longer.
- ❖ Add in the reserved meatballs, turn the heat to simmer and continue to cook for 6 to 7 minutes.
- ❖ Storing
- ❖ Place the meatballs in airtight containers or Ziploc bags; keep in your refrigerator for up to 3 to 4 days.
- ❖ Freeze the meatballs in airtight containers or heavy-duty freezer bags. Freeze up to 3 to 4 months. To defrost, slowly reheat in a saucepan. Bon appétit!

Nutrition: 252 Calories; 9.7g Fat; 5.3g Carbs; 34.2g Protein; 1.4g Fiber

Sides & Appetizers Recipes

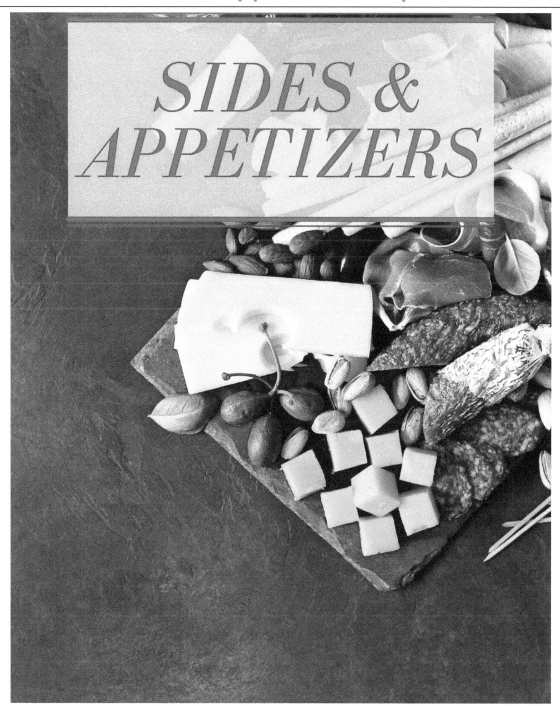

191) SPECIAL BRAISED ARTICHOKES

Cooking Time: 30 Minutes   **Servings:** 6

- ✓ ½ tsp salt
- ✓ 1½ pounds tomatoes, seeded and diced
- ✓ ½ cup almonds, toasted and sliced

Directions:

- ❖ Heat oil in a skillet over medium heat.
- ❖ Add artichokes, garlic, and lemon juice, and allow the garlic to sizzle.
- ❖ Season with salt.
- ❖ Reduce heat to medium-low, cover, and simmer for about 15 minutes.
- ❖ Uncover, add tomatoes, and simmer for another 10 minutes until the tomato liquid has mostly evaporated.
- ❖ Season with more salt and pepper.
- ❖ Sprinkle with toasted almonds.
- ❖ Enjoy!

Nutrition: Calories: 265, Total Fat: 1g, Saturated Fat: 2.6 g, Cholesterol: 0 mg, Sodium: 265 mg, Total Carbohydrate: 23 g, Dietary Fiber: 8.1 g, Total Sugars: 12.4 g, Protein: 7 g, Vitamin D: 0 mcg, Calcium: 81 mg, Iron: 2 mg, Potassium: 1077 mg

192) DELICIOUS FRIED GREEN BEANS

Cooking Time: 15 Minutes   **Servings:** 2

- ✓ 2 tbsp parmesan cheese
- ✓ ½ tsp garlic powder
- ✓ sea salt or plain salt
- ✓ freshly ground black pepper

Directions:

- ❖ Start by beating the egg and olive oil in a bowl.
- ❖ Then, mix the remaining Ingredients: in a separate bowl and set aside.
- ❖ Now, dip the green beans in the egg mixture and then coat with the dry mix.
- ❖ Finally, grease a baking pan, then transfer the beans to the pan and bake at 5 degrees F for about 12-15 minutes or until crisp.
- ❖ Serve warm.

Nutrition: Calories: 334, Total Fat: 23 g, Saturated Fat: 8.3 g, Cholesterol: 109 mg, Sodium: 397 mg, Total Carbohydrate: 10.9 g, Dietary Fiber: 4.3 g, Total Sugars: 1.9 g, Protein: 18.1 g, Vitamin D: 8 mcg, Calcium: 398 mg, Iron: 2 mg, Potassium: 274 mg

193) VEGGIE MEDITERRANEAN-STYLE PASTA

Cooking Time: 2 Hours   **Servings:** 4

- ✓ ½ tsp salt
- ✓ ½ tsp brown sugar
- ✓ freshly ground black pepper
- ✓ 1 piece aubergine
- ✓ 2 pieces courgettes
- ✓ 2 pieces red peppers, de-seeded
- ✓ 2 garlic cloves, peeled
- ✓ 2-3 tbsp olive oil
- ✓ 12 small vine-ripened tomatoes
- ✓ 16 ounces of pasta of your preferred shape, such as Gigli, conchiglie, etc.
- ✓ 3½ ounces parmesan cheese

Directions:

- ❖ Heat oil in a pan over medium heat.
- ❖ Add onions and fry them until tender.
- ❖ Add garlic and stir-fry for 1 minute.
- ❖ Add the remaining Ingredients: listed under the sauce and bring to a boil.
- ❖ Reduce the heat, cover, and simmer for 60 minutes.
- ❖ Season with black pepper and salt as needed. Set aside.
- ❖ Preheat oven to 350 degrees F.
- ❖ Chop up courgettes, aubergine and red peppers into 1-inch pieces.
- ❖ Place them on a roasting pan along with whole garlic cloves.
- ❖ Drizzle with olive oil and season with salt and black pepper.
- ❖ Mix the veggies well and roast in the oven for 45 minutes until they are tender.
- ❖ Add tomatoes just before 20 minutes to end time.
- ❖ Cook your pasta according to package instructions.
- ❖ Drain well and stir into the sauce.
- ❖ Divide the pasta sauce between 4 containers and top with vegetables.
- ❖ Grate some parmesan cheese on top and serve with bread.
- ❖ Enjoy!

Nutrition: Calories: 211, Total Fat: 14.9 g, Saturated Fat: 2.1 g, Cholesterol: 0 mg, Sodium: 317 mg, Total Carbohydrate: 20.1 g, Dietary Fiber: 5.7 g, Total Sugars: 11.7 g, Protein: 4.2 g, Vitamin D: 0 mcg, Calcium: 66 mg, Iron: 2 mg, Potassium: 955 mg

194) CLASSIC BASIL PASTA

Cooking Time: 40 Minutes   **Servings: 4**

Ingredients:

- ✓ 2 red peppers, de-seeded and cut into chunks
- ✓ 2 red onions cut into wedges
- ✓ 2 mild red chilies, de-seeded and diced
- ✓ 3 garlic cloves, coarsely chopped
- ✓ 1 tsp golden caster sugar
- ✓ 2 tbsp olive oil, plus extra for serving
- ✓ 2 pounds small ripe tomatoes, quartered
- ✓ 12 ounces pasta
- ✓ a handful of basil leaves, torn
- ✓ 2 tbsp grated parmesan
- ✓ salt
- ✓ pepper

Directions:

- ❖ Preheat oven to 390 degrees F.
- ❖ On a large roasting pan, spread peppers, red onion, garlic, and chilies.
- ❖ Sprinkle sugar on top.
- ❖ Drizzle olive oil and season with salt and pepper.
- ❖ Roast the veggies for 1minutes.
- ❖ Add tomatoes and roast for another 15 minutes.
- ❖ In a large pot, cook your pasta in salted boiling water according to instructions.
- ❖ Once ready, drain pasta.
- ❖ Remove the veggies from the oven and carefully add pasta.
- ❖ Toss everything well and let it cool.
- ❖ Spread over the containers.
- ❖ Before eating, place torn basil leaves on top, and sprinkle with parmesan.
- ❖ Enjoy!

Nutrition: Calories: 384, Total Fat: 10.8 g, Saturated Fat: 2.3 g, Cholesterol: 67 mg, Sodium: 133 mg, Total Carbohydrate: 59.4 g, Dietary Fiber: 2.3 g, Total Sugars: 5.7 g, Protein: 1 g, Vitamin D: 0 mcg, Calcium: 105 mg, Iron: 4 mg, Potassium: 422 mg

195) ORIGINAL RED ONION KALE PASTA

Cooking Time: 25 Minutes   **Servings: 4**

Ingredients:

- ✓ 2½ cups vegetable broth
- ✓ ¾ cup dry lentils
- ✓ ½ tsp of salt
- ✓ 1 bay leaf
- ✓ ¼ cup olive oil
- ✓ 1 large red onion, chopped
- ✓ 1 tsp fresh thyme, chopped
- ✓ ½ tsp fresh oregano, chopped
- ✓ 1 tsp salt, divided
- ✓ ½ tsp black pepper
- ✓ 8 ounces vegan sausage, sliced into ¼-inch slices
- ✓ 1 bunch kale, stems removed and coarsely chopped
- ✓ 1 pack rotini

Directions:

- ❖ Add vegetable broth, ½ tsp of salt, bay leaf, and lentils to a saucepan over high heat and bring to a boil.
- ❖ Reduce the heat to medium-low and allow to cook for about minutes until tender.
- ❖ Discard the bay leaf.
- ❖ Take another skillet and heat olive oil over medium-high heat.
- ❖ Stir in thyme, onions, oregano, ½ a tsp of salt, and pepper; cook for 1 minute.
- ❖ Add sausage and reduce heat to medium-low.
- ❖ Cook for 10 minutes until the onions are tender.
- ❖ Bring water to a boil in a large pot, and then add rotini pasta and kale.
- ❖ Cook for about 8 minutes until al dente.
- ❖ Remove a bit of the cooking water and put it to the side.
- ❖ Drain the pasta and kale and return to the pot.
- ❖ Stir in both the lentils mixture and the onions mixture.
- ❖ Add the reserved cooking liquid to add just a bit of moistness.
- ❖ Spread over containers.

Nutrition: Calories: 508, Total Fat: 17 g, Saturated Fat: 3 g, Cholesterol: 0 mg, Sodium: 2431 mg, Total Carbohydrate: 59.3 g, Dietary Fiber: 6 g, Total Sugars: 4.8 g, Protein: 30.9 g, Vitamin D: 0 mcg, Calcium: 256 mg, Iron: 8 mg, Potassium: 1686 mg

196) TUSCAN BAKED MUSHROOMS

Cooking Time: 20 Minutes   **Servings: 2**

Ingredients:

- ✓ ½ pound mushrooms (sliced)
- ✓ 2 tbsp olive oil (onion and garlic flavored)
- ✓ 1 can tomatoes
- ✓ 1 cup Parmesan cheese
- ✓ ½ tsp oregano
- ✓ 1 tbsp basil
- ✓ sea salt or plain salt
- ✓ freshly ground black pepper

Directions:

- ❖ Heat the olive oil in the pan and add the mushrooms, salt, and pepper. Cook for about 2 minutes.
- ❖ Then, transfer the mushrooms into a baking dish.
- ❖ Now, in a separate bowl mix the tomatoes, basil, oregano, salt, and pepper, and layer it on the mushrooms. Top it with Parmesan cheese.
- ❖ Finally, bake the dish at 0 degrees F for about 18-22 minutes or until done.
- ❖ Serve warm.

Nutrition: Calories: 358, Total Fat: 27 g, Saturated Fat: 10.2 g, Cholesterol: 40 mg, Sodium: 535 mg, Total Carbohydrate: 13 g, Dietary Fiber: 3.5 g, Total Sugars: 6.7 g, Protein: 23.2 g, Vitamin D: 408 mcg, Calcium: 526 mg, Iron: 4 mg, Potassium: 797 mg

197) TYPICAL MINT TABBOULEH

Cooking Time: 15 Minutes   **Servings: 6**

Ingredients:

- ✓ ¼ cup fine bulgur
- ✓ 1/3 cup water, boiling
- ✓ 3 tbsp lemon juice
- ✓ ¼ tsp honey
- ✓ 1 1/3 cups pistachios, finely chopped
- ✓ 1 cup curly parsley, finely chopped
- ✓ 1 small cucumber, finely chopped
- ✓ 1 medium tomato, finely chopped
- ✓ 4 green onions, finely chopped
- ✓ 1/3 cup fresh mint, finely chopped
- ✓ 3 tbsp olive oil

Directions:

- ❖ Take a large bowl and add bulgur and 3 cup of boiling water.
- ❖ Allow it to stand for about 5 minutes.
- ❖ Stir in honey and lemon juice and allow it to stand for 5 minutes more.
- ❖ Fluff up the bulgur with a fork and stir in the rest of the Ingredients.
- ❖ Season with salt and pepper.
- ❖ Enjoy!

Nutrition: Calories: 15 Total Fat: 13.5 g, Saturated Fat: 1.8 g, Cholesterol: 0 mg, Sodium: 78 mg, Total Carbohydrate: 9.2 g, Dietary Fiber: 2.8 g, Total Sugars: 2.9 g, Protein: 3.8 g, Vitamin D: 0 mcg, Calcium: 46 mg, Iron: 2 mg, Potassium: 359 mg

198) Italian Chicken Bacon Pasta

Cooking Time: 35 Minutes   **Servings: 4**

Ingredients:

- ✓ 8 ounces linguine pasta
- ✓ 3 slices of bacon
- ✓ 1 pound boneless chicken breast, cooked and diced
- ✓ Salt
- ✓ 1 6-ounce can artichoke hearts
- ✓ 2 ounce can diced tomatoes, undrained
- ✓ ¼ tsp dried rosemary
- ✓ 1/3 cup crumbled feta cheese, plus extra for topping
- ✓ 2/3 cup pitted black olives

Directions:

- ❖ Fill a large pot with salted water and bring to a boil.
- ❖ Add linguine and cook for 8-10 minutes until al dente.
- ❖ Cook bacon until brown, and then crumble.
- ❖ Season chicken with salt.
- ❖ Place chicken and bacon into a large skillet.
- ❖ Add tomatoes and rosemary and simmer the mixture for about 20 minutes.
- ❖ Stir in feta cheese, artichoke hearts, and olives, and cook until thoroughly heated.
- ❖ Toss the freshly cooked pasta with chicken mixture and cool.
- ❖ Spread over the containers.
- ❖ Before eating, garnish with extra feta if your heart desires!

Nutrition: 755, Total Fat: 22.5 g, Saturated Fat: 6.5 g, Cholesterol: 128 mg, Sodium: 852 mg, Total Carbohydrate: 75.4 g, Dietary Fiber: 7.3 g, Total Sugars: 3.4 g, Protein: 55.6 g, Vitamin D: 0 mcg, Calcium: 162 mg, Iron: 7 mg, Potassium: 524 mg

199)   LOVELY CREAMY GARLIC SHRIMP PASTA

Cooking Time: 15 Minutes   **Servings: 4**

Ingredients:

- ✓ 6 ounces whole-wheat spaghetti, your favorite
- ✓ 12 ounces raw shrimp, peeled, deveined, and cut into 1-inch pieces
- ✓ 1 bunch asparagus, trimmed and thinly sliced
- ✓ 1 large bell pepper, thinly sliced
- ✓ 3 cloves garlic, chopped
- ✓ 1¼ tsp kosher salt
- ✓ 1½ cups non-fat plain yogurt
- ✓ ¼ cup flat-leaf parsley, chopped
- ✓ 3 tbsp lemon juice
- ✓ 1 tbsp extra virgin olive oil
- ✓ ½ tsp fresh ground black pepper
- ✓ ¼ cup toasted pine nuts

Directions:

- ❖ Bring water to a boil in a large pot.
- ❖ Add spaghetti and cook for about minutes less than called for by the package instructions.
- ❖ Add shrimp, bell pepper, asparagus and cook for about 2-4 minutes until the shrimp are tender.
- ❖ Drain the pasta.
- ❖ In a large bowl, mash the garlic until paste forms.
- ❖ Whisk yogurt, parsley, oil, pepper, and lemon juice into the garlic paste.
- ❖ Add pasta mixture and toss well.
- ❖ Cool and spread over the containers.
- ❖ Sprinkle with pine nuts.
- ❖ Enjoy!

Nutrition: 504, Total Fat: 15.4 g, Saturated Fat: 4.9 g, Cholesterol: 199 mg, Sodium: 2052 mg, Total Carbohydrate: 42.2 g, Dietary Fiber: 3.5 g, Total Sugars: 26.6 g, Protein: 43.2 g, Vitamin D: 0 mcg, Calcium: 723 mg, Iron: 3 mg, Potassium: 3 mg

200)   Original Lemon Garlic Sardine Fettuccine

Cooking Time: 15 Minutes   **Servings: 4**

Ingredients:

- ✓ 8 ounces whole-wheat fettuccine
- ✓ 4 tbsp extra-virgin olive oil, divided
- ✓ 4 cloves garlic, minced
- ✓ 1 cup fresh breadcrumbs
- ✓ ¼ cup lemon juice
- ✓ 1 tsp freshly ground pepper
- ✓ ½ tsp of salt
- ✓ 2 4-ounce cans boneless and skinless sardines, dipped in tomato sauce
- ✓ ½ cup fresh parsley, chopped
- ✓ ¼ cup finely shredded parmesan cheese

Directions:

- ❖ Fill a large pot with water and bring to a boil.
- ❖ Cook pasta according to package instructions until tender (about 10 minutes).
- ❖ In a small skillet, heat 2 tbsp of oil over medium heat.
- ❖ Add garlic and cook for about 20 seconds, until sizzling and fragrant.
- ❖ Transfer the garlic to a large bowl.
- ❖ Add the remaining 2 tbsp of oil to skillet and heat over medium heat.
- ❖ Add breadcrumbs and cook for 5-6 minutes until golden and crispy.
- ❖ Whisk lemon juice, salt, and pepper into the garlic bowl.
- ❖ Add pasta to the garlic bowl, along with garlic, sardines, parmesan, and parsley; give it a gentle stir.
- ❖ Cool and spread over the containers.
- ❖ Before eating, sprinkle with breadcrumbs.
- ❖ Enjoy!

Nutrition: 633, Total Fat: 27.7 g, Saturated Fat: 6.4 g, Cholesterol: 40 mg, Sodium: 771 mg, Total Carbohydrate: 55.9 g, Dietary Fiber: 7.7 g, Total Sugars: 2.1 g, Protein: 38.6 g, Vitamin D: 0 mcg, Calcium: 274 mg, Iron: 7 mg, Potassium: mg

201)   DELICIOUS SPINACH ALMOND STIR-FRY

Cooking Time: 10 Minutes   **Servings: 2**

Ingredients:

- ✓ 2 ounces spinach
- ✓ 1 tbsp coconut oil
- ✓ 3 tbsp almond, slices
- ✓ sea salt or plain salt
- ✓ freshly ground black pepper

Directions:

- ❖ Start by heating a skillet with coconut oil; add spinach and let it cook.
- ❖ Then, add salt and pepper as the spinach is cooking.
- ❖ Finally, add in the almond slices.
- ❖ Serve warm.

Nutrition: 117, Total Fat: 11.4 g, Saturated Fat: 6.2 g, Cholesterol: 0 mg, Sodium: 23 mg, Total Carbohydrate: 2.9 g, Dietary Fiber: 1.7 g, Total Sugars: 0.g, Protein: 2.7 g, Vitamin D: 0 mcg, Calcium: 52 mg, Iron: 1 mg, Potassium: 224 mg

202) **ITALIAN BBQ CARROTS**

Cooking Time: 30 Minutes   **Servings:** 8

Ingredients:

- ✓ 2 pounds baby carrots (organic)
- ✓ 1 tbsp olive oil
- ✓ 1 tbsp garlic powder
- ✓ 1 tbsp onion powder
- ✓ sea salt or plain salt
- ✓ freshly ground black pepper

Directions:

- ❖ Mix all the Ingredients: in a plastic bag so that the carrots are well coated with the mixture.
- ❖ Then, on the BBQ grill place a piece of aluminum foil and spread the carrots in a single layer.
- ❖ Finally, grill for 30 minutes or until tender.
- ❖ Serve warm.

Nutrition: 388, Total Fat: 1.9 g, Saturated Fat: 0.3 g, Cholesterol: 0 mg, Sodium: 89 mg, Total Carbohydrate: 10.8 g, Dietary Fiber: 3.4 g, Total Sugars: 6 g, Protein: 1 g, Vitamin D: 0 mcg, Calcium: 40 mg, Iron: 1 mg, Potassium: 288 mg

203) **MEDITERRANEAN-STYLE BAKED ZUCCHINI STICKS**

Cooking Time: 20 Minutes   **Servings:** 8

Ingredients:

- ✓ ¼ cup feta cheese, crumbled
- ✓ 4 zucchini
- ✓ ¼ cup parsley, chopped
- ✓ ½ cup tomatoes, minced
- ✓ ½ cup kalamata olives, pitted and minced
- ✓ 1 cup red bell pepper, minced
- ✓ 1 tbsp oregano
- ✓ ¼ cup garlic, minced
- ✓ 1 tbsp basil
- ✓ sea salt or plain salt
- ✓ freshly ground black pepper

Directions:

- ❖ Start by cutting zucchini in half (lengthwise) and scoop out the middle.
- ❖ Then, combine garlic, black pepper, bell pepper, oregano, basil, tomatoes, and olives in a bowl.
- ❖ Now, fill in the middle of each zucchini with this mixture. Place these on a prepared baking dish and bake the dish at 0 degrees F for about 15 minutes.
- ❖ Finally, top with feta cheese and broil on high for 3 minutes or until done. Garnish with parsley.
- ❖ Serve warm.

Nutrition: 53, Total Fat: 2.2 g, Saturated Fat: 0.9 g, Cholesterol: 4 mg, Sodium: 138 mg, Total Carbohydrate: 7.5 g, Dietary Fiber: 2.1 g, Total Sugars: 3 g, Protein: 2.g, Vitamin D: 0 mcg, Calcium: 67 mg, Iron: 1 mg, Potassium: 353 mg

204) **ARTICHOKE OLIVE PASTA**

Cooking Time: 25 Minutes   **Servings:** 4

Ingredients:

- ✓ salt
- ✓ pepper
- ✓ 2 tbsp olive oil, divided
- ✓ 2 garlic cloves, thinly sliced
- ✓ 1 can artichoke hearts, drained, rinsed, and quartered lengthwise
- ✓ 1-pint grape tomatoes, halved lengthwise, divided
- ✓ ½ cup fresh basil leaves, torn apart
- ✓ 12 ounces whole-wheat spaghetti
- ✓ ½ medium onion, thinly sliced
- ✓ ½ cup dry white wine
- ✓ 1/3 cup pitted Kalamata olives, quartered lengthwise
- ✓ ¼ cup grated Parmesan cheese, plus extra for serving

Directions:

- ❖ Fill a large pot with salted water.
- ❖ Pour the water to a boil and cook your pasta according to package instructions until al dente.
- ❖ Drain the pasta and reserve 1 cup of the cooking water.
- ❖ Return the pasta to the pot and set aside.
- ❖ Heat 1 tbsp of olive oil in a large skillet over medium-high heat.
- ❖ Add onion and garlic, season with pepper and salt, and cook well for about 3-4 minutes until nicely browned.
- ❖ Add wine and cook for 2 minutes until evaporated.
- ❖ Stir in artichokes and keep cooking 2-3 minutes until brown.
- ❖ Add olives and half of your tomatoes.
- ❖ Cook well for 1-2 minutes until the tomatoes start to break down.
- ❖ Add pasta to the skillet.
- ❖ Stir in the rest of the tomatoes, cheese, basil, and remaining oil.
- ❖ Thin the mixture with the reserved pasta water if needed.
- ❖ Place in containers and sprinkle with extra cheese.
- ❖ Enjoy!

Nutrition: 340, Total Fat: 11.9 g, Saturated Fat: 3.3 g, Cholesterol: 10 mg, Sodium: 278 mg, Total Carbohydrate: 35.8 g, Dietary Fiber: 7.8 g, Total Sugars: 4.8 g, Protein: 11.6 g, Vitamin D: 0 mcg, Calcium: 193 mg, Iron: 3 mg, Potassium: 524 mg

CONCLUSIONS

Your Mediterranean Diet Cookbook is coming to an end, but don't worry. You can keep using the cheat sheets and recipes in this book for a lifetime! This cookbook is full of delicious Mediterranean dishes that will help you lose weight, feel healthier, and live longer.

In this cookbook, you'll find healthy Mediterranean recipes that are designed to be easy to make. Our recipes can be made from scratch at home or from a pre-made frozen meal or pre-packaged product. Look for our handy tips at the end of each recipe, as well as our tips and tricks for making the best dishes every time. Use them to your advantage and make all your favorite dishes better than ever!

You found a quick overview of the Mediterranean diet, healthy eating tips, and recipes designed to help anyone start an effort to lose weight and improve overall health.

The Mediterranean diet is a healthy way to eat.

Does the Mediterranean diet agree with your medical history? E.g., Crohn's disease, colitis, or intestinal problems? If yes, then the Mediterranean Diet may be proper for you...The fiber found in all fruits and vegetables is beneficial to the digestive system and a great energy source. Last but not least, antioxidants help prevent free radicals from causing cell damage.

The Mediterranean diet has been trending among people in recent years, and it seems that more and more people are trying to follow this regimen.

However, before you start following the Mediterranean diet or any other diet for that matter, you need to understand what the Mediterranean diet is all about. Adopting this type of diet can help you gain many weight loss benefits compared to eating a typical Western diet.

I hope now you understand how easy it is to adopt this type of diet as long as you maintain your basic requirements. The daily intake of fresh produce, meat, and seafood and the daily dose of high-quality fats can help you achieve success in your efforts to control your health and fitness goals by using this diet as a guide.

Alexander Sandler

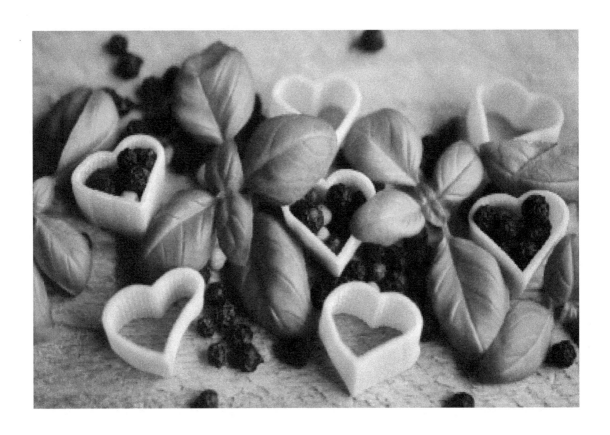

AUTHOR BIBLIOGRAPHY

THE MEDITERRANEAN DIET: *Cookbook for Beginners: Master Guidance, and More than 100 Recipes to Get You Started.*

THE MEDITERRANEAN DIET FOR BEGINNERS: *The Complete Guide with More than 100 Delicious Recipes, and Tips for Success!*

THE MEDITERRANEAN DIET COOKBOOK: *A Guide for Beginners: Discover 100+ Delicious Recipes for Healthy Eating. Enjoy your Food Every Day!!!*

THE MEDITERRANEAN DIET COPLETE GUIDE FOR BEGINNER: *2 Books in 1: The Ultimate Guide for Beginners: Discover 200+ Delicious Recipes and Start to Lose Weight for a Healthy Eating! Enjoy your Food Every Day!!!*

THE MEDITERRANEAN DIET FOR VEGETARIANS: *Complete Guide and More than 100 Delicious Mediterranean recipes suitable for Vegetarians*

THE MEDITERRANEAN & KETO DIET: *The Guide on the Combination of the Mediterranean Diet and the Keto Diet to boost your weight loss and Get Fit and Healthy! Cookbook for Beginners: Master Guidance, and More than 150 Recipes to Get You Started! 4-week Meal Plan Included*

THE MEDITERRANEAN DIET SPECIAL EDITION: *4 Books in 1: A Simple Guide to Start the Mediterranean Diet suitable for Vegetarian and Athlete with more 400+ Recipes! 4-Week Keto Meal Plan Included! Start to be Healthy and Fit!*

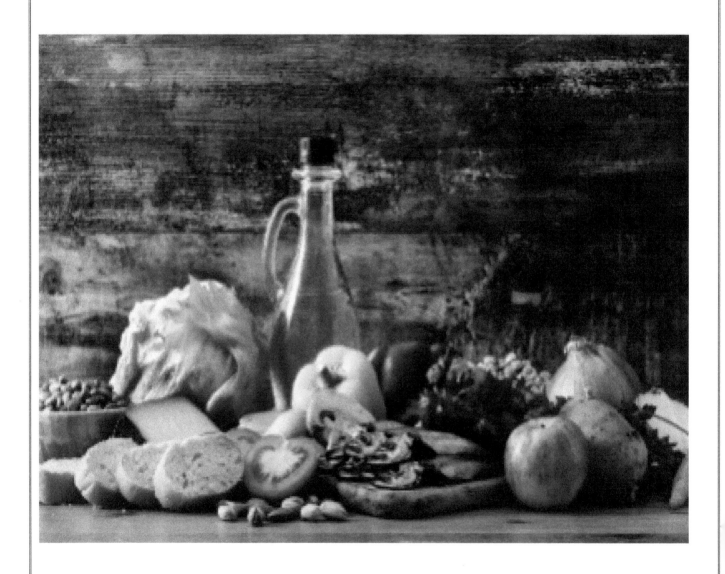

CONCLUSIONS

The Mediterranean diet emphasizes fresh foods such as fruits and vegetables in combination with whole grains. It is low in red meat and high in fish, poultry, nuts, and beans. This diet has many different types of food groups to help you bring variety into your day: bread (whole grain), beans/lentils/nuts/seeds, berries/vegetables, dairy (low fat), olive oil, refrigerated or uncooked fish/meat (preferably fatty fish), unlimited wine and alcohol (usually no more than one glass per day), cheese (low fat), fruit (fresh), eggplant, potatoes (unpeeled), cabbage (raw), and pasta (whole grain). Add other vegetables to meals, such as tomatoes. Don't overcook the meat. All meats should be grilled or broiled over a low flame that does not brown the meat to reduce cancer risk. It is best to use steaks instead of hamburgers or ground beef. Make sure poultry is white meat from chicken or turkey, not dark meat, including liver or bones. Use lean cuts of beef/pork such as round steak or tenderloin instead of fattier cuts such as sirloin or rib-eye steaks. Fish should be firm-fleshed and skin-on and fried in relatively light oil such as olive oil instead of butter or margarine, as this can increase the number of calories you eat per serving. Always use white meat turkey instead of dark meat breast for recipes that call for one type of meat since white meat has less fat: per serving than dark meat chicken breast. All fruits should be eaten raw to provide taste plus their vitamin content, including vitamin C plus others. Mediterranean health is a healthy lifestyle that includes eating lots of fresh fruits, lots of vegetables, whole grains, healthy fats, moderate amounts of alcohol, seafood, poultry, and engaging in physical activity. The Mediterranean diet is a healthy eating pattern recommended for people living in northern climates who are at low risk of developing cardiovascular disease or diabetes. It is called the Mediterranean diet because it originated in Greece, Turkey, and the Mediterranean Sea's southern countries. These countries (and others in the region) share many cultural and culinary similarities.

The Mediterranean diet, often called the Mediterranean lifestyle, has been getting a lot of hype lately. More and more people are trying to eat healthier or simply starting to think about what they eat. Mediterranean diets, sometimes called the traditional Mediterranean diet or traditional lifestyle was initially designed for those who worked on farms. They contain foods that lead to healthy hearts and muscular bodies. Many call the Mediterranean diet a "bikini-body diet." As surprising as it may be, there is not much difference between the Mediterranean diet and the Atkins diet. All three focus on eating healthy foods. The Mediterranean diet is based on the fact that food often contains more than one nutrient. Most fruits and vegetables have some fat: or sugar in them. The idea is to eat various foods from all parts of the world, which includes different types of meats, cheeses, grains, legumes, nuts, and other foods. In addition to being a great way to eat well naturally, the Mediterranean diet is good for your health. It has been shown to help with weight loss and cardiovascular disease prevention. It also promotes weight maintenance after weight loss. Studies have shown that it can reduce cholesterol levels in obese people and reduce blood pressure in people with hypertension. People with high cholesterol can have their grades lowered by following a Mediterranean diet. Studies have also shown that it can help fight cancer naturally, causing tumors to shrink faster than other dietary regimens.

Alexander Sandler

CPSIA information can be obtained
at www.ICGtesting.com
Printed in the USA
LVHW062103250521
688445LV00011B/1106

9 781802 538076